D1758712

Donated to GRH Library
by Robin Youngs 4.11.2015

Manual of

Head and Neck
Surgical Oncology

Manual of

Head and Neck Surgical Oncology

Edited by

Nicholas Stafford MB ChB, FRCS
Professor, ENT and Head and Neck Surgery
Hull York Medical School
University of Hull
Hull, UK

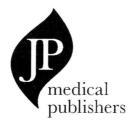

JP
medical
publishers

London • Philadelphia • Panama City • New Delhi

ISBN: 978-1-907816-69-7

British Library Cataloguing in Publication Data
A catalogue record for this book is available from the British Library

Library of Congress Cataloging in Publication Data
A catalog record for this book is available from the Library of Congress

Publisher: Geoff Greenwood
Development Editor: Gavin Smith
Editorial Assistant: Katie Pattullo
Design: Designers Collective Ltd

Preface

From the outset of their career, surgical trainees involved in head and neck surgery have a number of significant issues to contend with. One of these is the diversity and complexity of the topic, both clinical and anatomical. Another is that head and neck surgery often occupies a relatively peripheral position of importance in the context of their primary specialty. Looked at another way, most ENT, plastic and maxillofacial surgeons do not end up working in head and neck oncology once they move on to more senior surgical positions.

Given the above, it can be difficult to justify spending an inordinate amount of time reviewing the many excellent but necessarily lengthy books on the topic. However, trainees still need to understand and be able to practice the fundamentals of this particular surgical craft. The purpose of *Manual of Head and Neck Surgical Oncology* is to allow the junior doctor to do exactly that, and to be able to demonstrate an understanding of what is involved in performing most of the standard major head and neck procedures.

The book is not intended to provide comprehensive coverage of the various tumors encountered in the region: the authors presuppose a basic knowledge of relevant etiology, anatomy, clinical features, histopathological patterns, and detailed treatment options and their execution. The book has been written more as an 'aide-memoire', highlighting important anatomical points and the order of events in a number of set-piece surgical procedures. The intention is to provide the trainee with a practical guide to the incremental surgical steps that need to be undertaken to successfully complete these procedures. Hopefully, using this book as a guide, he or she can quickly and easily refresh their memory of what is involved in such procedures so that when a senior colleague invites them to carry out the operation they are not filled with fear. Instead they will be able to display their sound knowledge of what they are expected to do and how they should do it.

Nicholas Stafford
July 2015

Contents

Contributors

Mymoona Alzouebi MRCP, MSC, FRCR
Consultant Clinical Oncologist
Weston Park Hospital
Sheffield Teaching Hospital NHS
Foundation Trust
Sheffield, UK

Simon D Carr BSc(Hons), MD, FRCS
ENT Specialist Registrar
Royal Hallamshire Hospital
Sheffield, UK

Stephen Crank FDSRCS(Ed), FRCS(Max Fac)
Consultant Maxillofacial, Head and
Neck Surgeon
Department of Oral and
Maxillofacial Surgery
Hull and East Yorkshire NHS Trust
Hull, UK

R James A England MB ChB, FRCS(ORL-HNS)
Consultant ENT/Thyroid Surgeon
Department of Otolaryngology, Head and
Neck Surgery
Hull and East Yorkshire Hospitals Trust
East Yorkshire, UK

Terry M Jones, BSc(Hons), FRCSEd, FRCS(ORL-HNS), MD, FHEA, FASE(RCS)
Professor of Head and Neck Surgery
Department of Molecular and Clinical
Cancer Medicine
Institute of Translational Medicine
University of Liverpool
Liverpool, UK

Tristram Lesser AKC, FRCSEd, MS
ENT and Skull Base Surgeon
Skull Base Service
Department of ENT Head and
Neck Surgery
Aintree University Hospital
Liverpool, UK

Paolo Matteucci Mb ChB, MRCS (Ed), FRCS (Plast)
Consultant Plastic, Reconstructive and
Head and Neck Surgeon
Department of Plastic and
Reconstructive Surgery
Castle Hill Hospital
Honorary Senior Clinical Lecturer
Hull York Medical School
Hull, UK

Bruce Mathew MBChB, FRCS(Ed)SN, ChM
Consultant Neurosurgeon
Department of Neurosurgery
Hull Royal Infirmary
Hull, UK

Elizabeth Nelson BSc, MSc, RCSLT, HCPC
Principal Speech and Language Therapist
(Macmillan)
Speech and Language Therapy Department
Hull Royal Infirmary
Hull, UK

Ashis Pathak MBBS, MS (Gen Surg), MCh (Neurosurg), MNAMS, FICS
Director of Neurosurgery
Fortis Hospital
Mohali, India

Narayanan Prepageran FRCSEd
Professor of Otorhinolaryngology Head
and Neck Surgery
Department of Otorhinolaryngology,
Head and Neck Surgery
University of Malaya Medical Center
Kuala Lumpur, Malaysia

Martin H Robinson MB, BCh, FRCP, FRCR, MD, Cert APS
Consultant Clinical Oncologist
University of Sheffield
Sheffield Teaching Hospitals
Foundation Trust
Sheffield, UK

David R Salvage BSc, MBBS, FRCS,FRCR
Consultant Radiologist
Department of Radiology
Hull Royal Infirmary
Hull, UK

Richard J Shaw MD, FRCS(OMFS), FDS, MBChB(Hons), BDS, PGCert
Professor of Head and Neck Surgery
Honorary Consultant in Oral and
Maxillofacial, Head and Neck Surgery
Department of Molecular and Clinical
Cancer Medicine
North West Cancer Research Centre
Regional Maxillofacial Unit
Aintree University Hospitals NHS
Foundation Trust
Associate Director of NIHR Clinical
Research Network (Cancer)
National Institute of Health Research
Liverpool, UK

Ruth A Simpson BSc Hons (Nutrition and Dietetics)
Macmillan Highly Specialist Head and
Neck Dietitian
Department of Nutrition and Dietetics
Hull and East Yorkshire Hospitals
Hull, UK

Nicholas Stafford MB ChB, FRCS
Professor, ENT and Head and Neck Surgery
Hull York Medical School
University of Hull
Hull, UK

Ing Ping Tang MS, ORL-HNS
Consultant ENT Surgeon
Faculty of Medicine
University of Malaysia Sarawak
Sarawak, Malaysia

John Waldron FRCS
Consultant Head and Neck Surgeon
Royal United Hospital
Bath, UK

Angela K Waweru MBChB, MRCP
Specialist Registrar in Clinical Oncology
Weston Park Hospital
Sheffield, UK

Liz K Wells MSc, PgDip, BSc Hons, RD
Advanced Research Dietitian
Hull York Medical School
University of Hull
Hull, UK

Robin Youngs MD, FRCS
Consultant Otolaryngologist
Department of Otolaryngology
Gloucestershire Hospitals NHS
Foundation Trust
Gloucester, UK

1 | Head and neck cancer: etiology and epidemiology

Simon Carr

Etiology

Tobacco and alcohol

Tobacco smoke has been identified as the main causative agent in head and neck squamous cell carcinoma (HNSCC) development with up to 98% of patients being smokers (Tuyns et al. 1988). Increased duration and intensity of smoking has been shown to increase the risk of developing HNSCC. Wynder et al. (1976) showed that the relative risk of developing laryngeal cancer from smoking 10 cigarettes per day was 4.4 compared with 34.4 for those that smoked 40 per day. The method of smoking also plays an important role, with cigars associated with a 10-fold increase and pipe smoking a 6- to 10-fold increase in cancer risk of the larynx and oropharynx combined.

La Vecchia et al. (1997) estimated that between 25% and 68% of HNSCC were attributable to ethanol consumption. While ethanol is not itself a carcinogen, it functions as a tumor promoter or cocarcinogen and when combined with tobacco, has been shown to act synergistically. Multiple mechanisms are involved in alcohol-associated HNSCC development including its local effects, the effect of acetaldehyde (AA), the first metabolite of ethanol oxidation, the induction of cytochrome P-4502E1 (CYP2E1) leading to the generation of reactive oxygen species, and enhanced procarcinogen activation, as well as the modulation of cellular regeneration and nutritional deficiencies.

Ethanol acts locally as a solvent, facilitating the penetration of carcinogenic compounds into the mucosa. Chronic alcoholism causes atrophy and lipomatous metamorphosis of the salivary gland parenchyma, leading to a reduction in saliva production. The mucosa surface is, therefore, inadequately rinsed and exposed to increased concentrations of carcinogens for a prolonged duration.

Studies have shown that AA is primarily responsible for the cocarcinogenic effect of ethanol. AA is formed during the metabolism of ethanol by alcohol dehydrogenase (ADH) and aldehyde dehydrogenase

(ALDH). Numerous in vitro and in vivo experiments have shown that AA has a direct mutagenic and carcinogenic effect, inducing inflammation and metaplasia of tracheal epithelium, delaying cell cycle progression and enhancing cell injury associated with hyper-regeneration. When inhaled, AA has been shown to cause nasopharyngeal and laryngeal carcinoma in a rat model. Genetic linkage studies in alcoholics have produced striking evidence about the causal role of AA and ethanol-associated HNSCC. Individuals who accumulate AA due to a polymorphism and/or a mutation in the gene coding for enzymes responsible for AA generation and detoxification have been shown to have an increased HNSCC risk. A comprehensive study of the ALDH2 genotype and cancer prevalence in a cohort of alcoholic patients in Japan showed that the frequency of inactive ALDH2 increased remarkably among alcoholics with HNSCC (Yokoyama et al. 1998).

Smoking and poor oral hygiene have been associated with an increase in AA levels in the oral cavity and pharynx. Smoking alters the flora from gram-negative to gram-positive bacteria and increases the levels of *Candida albicans,* both of which increase the levels of AA.

Chronic alcohol consumption leads to an induction of CYP2E1, which metabolizes ethanol to AA. This cytochrome enzyme is also involved in the metabolism of various xenobiotics, including procarcinogens. Induction of CYP2E1 in the upper aerodigestive tract may be particularly relevant with respect with respect to the procarcinogens present in tobacco smoke and the established synergism between them. In a meta-analysis, Tang et al. (2010) demonstrated an increased risk of developing HNSCC with the CYP2E1 polymorphisms PstI/RsaI (odds ratio 1.96) and DraI (odds ratio 1.56).

The type of alcoholic beverage consumed affects the risk of developing cancer. In a population study of 28,180, it was found that, compared with non-drinkers, subjects who drank 7–21 units of alcohol per week of beer and/or spirits, but no wine had an increased risk of developing oropharyngeal or esophageal cancer (relative risk 0.5). In those subjects that consumed over 21 units per week, their risk of developing cancer was higher compared to the group who drank 7–21 units in both the group that drank wine (relative risk 1.7) and those that did not (relative risk 5.2).

Viruses

Human papilloma virus (HPV) has been identified as a causative agent of HNSCC, in particular oropharyngeal SCC (Parkin 2011). The virus acts by infecting epithelial cells of mucosal surfaces, matching its own life cycle to that of the epithelial cells and replicating to produce new virus particles just as the cells become squamous and reach the surface of the mucosa.

The prevalence of HPV varies within the subsites of the head and neck region. According to two meta-analyses, the prevalence for all subsites combined is 25–28%, but for those in the oropharynx, the prevalence increases to approximately 40%.

Several subtypes are thought to be responsible and are stratified according to their risk: types 6, 11 (low risk), types 31, 33 (medium risk) and types 16, 18 (high risk). The prevalence of HPV-associated cancer quoted in the literature varies. Anwar et al. (1993) stated that approximately 25% of all laryngeal squamous cell carcinomas harbor HPV infection, but rates have been quoted as being as high as 35–60%. Epstein–Barr virus has been implicated in the development of nasopharyngeal cancer, most commonly non-keratinizing (differentiated) carcinoma (WHO type 2) and undifferentiated carcinoma (WHO type 3), which together account for 95% of cases in the Far East.

Dietary factors

Case control studies have shown up to an 80% reduction in cancer risk in people who have a high intake of fruit and vegetables. A high intake of red and processed meat has been associated with an increased risk of laryngeal cancer in case-control studies. In one study, it was demonstrated that those who consumed a western-style diet, high in fried, barbecued and processed meat, had an odds ratio of 3.2.

Many patients with HNSCC have a poor nutritional status, as a result of chronic alcoholism or caused directly by the tumor itself. Poor nutritional status may contribute to alcohol-associated carcinogenesis and is also associated with a poor prognosis.

A diet high in salt-cured fish and meat, typically consumed in areas of Asia, North Africa, and the Arctic is associated with nasopharyngeal carcinoma with odds ratios of 2.45 (95% CI: 2.03–2.94) and 2.09 (95% CI: 1.22–3.60), respectively, related to accumulation of carcinogenic nitrosamines. Conversely, a diet high in carotenoids has demonstrated a potential protective role against its development.

Occupational factors

Nickel and chromate refining workers have an increased incidence of laryngeal SCC. Exposure to coal dust has been shown to give a risk ratio of 6.0 with > 50 years exposure demonstrated to increase the risk by 3.6 times.

There is no general consensus as to whether asbestos exposure causes laryngeal cancer. A meta-analysis carried out in 1999 of asbestos-exposed cohort showed a 33–57% increase in the risk of developing laryngeal cancer (Goodman et al. 1999). However, other studies do not concur. Magnani et al. (2008) found that in a cohort of 3434 people, 16 developed laryngeal cancer compared to an expected value of 12.2, a non-significant difference. Another study found that asbestos exposure resulted in a non-significant odds ratio of 1.24 of developing laryngeal cancer subsequent to asbestos exposure.

Laryngopharyngeal reflux

Several studies including a meta-analysis by Qadeer et al. (2005) have demonstrated a causal relationship between laryngopharyngeal reflux and laryngeal cancer, while others have refuted this. Currently, there is no general consensus as to whether a link between laryngopharyngeal reflux and HNSCC exists.

Molecular and genetic factors

HNSCC arises from a common premalignant progenitor followed by outgrowth of clonal populations associated with cumulative genetic alterations and phenotypic progression to invasive malignancy (Califano et al. 1996). These genetic alterations result in inactivation of tumor suppressor genes and activation of proto-oncogenes by deletions, point mutations, promoter methylation, and gene amplification.

Epidermal growth factor receptor (EGFR) is a cell surface receptor for members of the epidermal factor family. EGFR dimerization stimulates its intrinsic intracellular protein – tyrosine kinase activity, which, in turn, causes increased activity in the downstream pathway. As EGFR is an important activator of mitogenic signaling; its increased activation leads to cellular proliferation. Overactivation of EGFR is well recognized in HNSCC and premalignant mucosa and occurs in up to 90% of cases (Grandis et al. 1993).

The phosphatidylinositide 3-kinase (P13K)/protein kinase B (AKT) pathway is an important downstream effector of the EGFR and its activation occurs in up to 90% of HNSCC cases. The tumor suppressor gene phosphatase and tensin homologue (*PTEN*) inhibits the P13/AKT pathway promoting G1 cell cycle arrest. Activation of the pathway may occur through several mechanisms including amplification of the PIK3CA locus (30–40% of cases), amplification of AKT (20–30% of cases) or methylation of the PTEN locus (Pedrero et al. 2005).

The most common genetic alterations are loss of heterozygosity (LOH) at chromosomal locations 9p, 3p, and 17p, as well as 5q, 8p, 9q, and 11p. LOH at 9p21 is an early event in HNSCC development and is found in 70–80% of cases. The CDKN2A gene locus found in chromosome 9p21 encodes p16[INK4A] and p14[ARF], which regulate the G1 cell cycle and are responsible for the MDM2 (murine double minute 2 protein)-mediated degradation of p53.

The tumor suppressor gene fragile histidine triad (*FIHT*) and ras-associated domain family member 1 (RASSF1A) are located at 3p14 and 3p21, respectively, and are associated with the development of HNSCC. These genes are inactivated by a combination of LOH of 3p that occurs in up to 70% of cases and hypermethylation of the normally unmethylated CpG islands of the gene promoter regions. The mechanisms by which inactivation of each of these tumor suppressor genes causes HNSCC remains unclear but it has been proposed that RASSF1A interacts with and stabilizes microtubule formation during mitosis.

LOH of 17p and point mutations of the p53 gene are seen in approximately 50% of cases, occurring late in the progression from epithelial dysplasia to invasive carcinoma. Amplification of 11q13 and overexpression of cyclin D1, which enables progression from G1 to S phase of the cell cycle through phosphorylation of the retinoblastoma (*Rb*) gene, is seen in 30–60% of HNSCC cases and is associated with an increased rate of lymph node metastases and poor prognosis. Several putative oncogenes are located in this area, including int-2 and hst-1, both members of the fibroblast growth factor family. The aberrant expression of the members of the ras and myc gene family, EGFR, Bcl-2 and Bax are believed to contribute toward cancer development (Ah-See et al. 1994).

Several genetic conditions are associated with an increased risk of HNSCC: Li-Fraumeni's syndrome is an autosomal dominant condition involving the mutation of p53 gene. Fanconi's anemia, Bloom's syndrome and ataxia-telangiectasia are autosomal recessive disorders associated with increased chromosomal fragility and cancer susceptibility.

Epidemiology

HNSCC encompasses malignancies of the oral cavity, nasopharynx, oropharynx, larynx, and hypopharynx. It accounted for 2.8/100,000 of all cancers in the United Kingdom in 2011 and represents the seventh most common cancer in Europe. HNSCC is the sixth most common form of cancer in the world with a global incidence of 700,000 cases per year. In the United Kingdom, laryngeal cancer is the largest subgroup of HNSCC, accounting for 50% of new cases. In 2008, there were 2300 new cases diagnosed, consisting of 1890 males and 402 females giving a male:female ratio of 5:1. The incidence rises sharply after the sixth decade with the zenith being at 75–79 years, resulting in 75% of cases being in those aged over 60 years (CRUK 2009).

An increased ratio of laryngeal cancer in males compared with females is reflected throughout Europe and Worldwide. In the United Kingdom, the male to female ratio is five compared to an average figure of nine in the countries making up the European Union. The variation in incidence rates between both countries, and between men and women, are likely to reflect the variations in the prevalence of smoking and to a slightly lesser extent alcohol consumption.

The most common laryngeal subsite for SCC, with 73% of cases, is the glottis, followed by the supraglottis with 24% and the subglottis with 3%. In an epidemiological study of 8987 patients with laryngeal cancer in South-East England, Coupland et al. (2009) found that a higher proportion of men presented with glottic cancer 42.4% versus 26.4%, whereas supraglottic cancer was more common in women 24.4% versus 14.2%.

Oral and oropharyngeal SCC represents 10–15% of all head and neck tumors. In 2004, there were 67,000 new cases of oropharyngeal cancer in the European Union. The incidence rates are higher in Western Europe, compared with Northern and Southern Europe. However, the highest mortality rates are reported in Eastern Europe. In the United Kingdom, there were 1346 new cases diagnosed in 2009 with numbers increasing since the late 1980s, particularly in men aged between 35 and 64. European age-standardized incidence rates have increased for men and women by 25% and 28%, respectively, a trend that has become increasingly apparent in young adults. Rates in Scotland are higher than in other parts of the United Kingdom for both men and women with a lifetime risk of 1.84% in males and 0.74% in females in Scotland compared to 1.06% and 0.48%, respectively, in the rest of the United Kingdom, possibly reflecting the increased tobacco and alcohol consumption among its population.

Hypopharyngeal cancer accounts for 3–5% of all HNSCC. Subsite variation exists within the hypopharynx with pyriform fossa being the most common (70%), followed by postcricoid (15%) and posterior pharyngeal wall (15%). Overall there is a male preponderance, but gender variation exists with a male prevalence in pyriform fossa and posterior pharyngeal wall and a female prevalence in postcricoid tumors. An incidence among males of 2.5/100,000 is seen in western and central Europe, India and Brazil and of 0.5/100,000 in northern Europe, eastern Asia and Africa.

Although uncommon in the United Kingdom with an incidence of 0.5/100,000, accounting for 1–2% of all HNSCC, nasopharyngeal carcinoma is endemic in Hong Kong and southern China with an incidence of 50/100,000 (Yu 1991).

Further reading

Ganly I, Patel SG. Epidemiology and prevention of head and neck cancer. In: Watkinson JC, Gilbert RW (eds), Stell and Maran's Textbook of Head and Neck Surgery and Oncology, 5th edn. London: Hodder Arnold, 2012.

Stafford ND. Aetiology of head and neck cancer. In: Gleeson M, Browning GG, Burton MJ, et al (eds), Scott-Brown's Otorhinolaryngology, Head and Neck Surgery, 7th edn. London: Hodder Arnold, 2008.

References

Ah-See KW, Cooke TG, Pickford IR, et al. An allelotype of squamous carcinoma of the head and neck using microsatellite markers. Cancer Res 1994; 54:1617–21.

Anwar K, Nakakuki K, Naiki H, Inuzuka M. Ras gene mutations and HPV infection are common in human laryngeal carcinoma. Int J Cancer 1993; 53:22–8.

Coupland VH, Chapman P, Linklater KM, et al. Trends in the epidemiology of larynx and lung cancer in South-East England, 1985–2004. Br J Cancer 2009; 100:167–9.

CRUK 2009. Laryngeal cancer – survival statistics [Online]. http://www.info.cancerresearch.org/cancerstats/types/larynx/survival. (Last accessed 15 October 2011.)

Goodman M, Morgan RW, Ray R, et al. Cancer in asbestos-exposed occupational cohorts: a meta-analysis. Cancer Causes Control 1999; 10:453–65.

Grandis JR, Tweardy DJ. Elevated levels of transforming growth factor alpha and epidermal growth factor receptor messenger RNA are early markers of carcinogenesis in head and neck cancer. Cancer Res 1993; 53:3579–84.

Magnani C, Ferrante D, Barone-Adesi F, et al. Cancer risk after cessation of asbestos exposure: a cohort of Italian asbestos cement workers. Occup Environ Med 2008; 65:164–70.

Pedrero JM, Carracedo DG, Pinto CM, et al. Frequent genetic and biochemical alterations of the PI 3-K/

AKT/PTEN pathway in head and neck squamous cell carcinoma. Int J Cancer 2005; 114:242–8.

Qadeer MA, Colabianchi N, Vaezi MF. Is GERD a risk factor for laryngeal cancer? Laryngoscope 2005; 115:486–91.

Tang K, Li Y, Zhang Z, et al. The PstI/RsaI and DraI polymorphisms of CYP2E1 and head and neck cancer risk: a meta-analysis based on 21 case-control studies. BMC Cancer 2010; 10:575.

Tuyns AJ, Esteve J, Raymond L, et al. Cancer of the larynx/hypopharynx, tobacco and alcohol: IARC international case-control study in Turin and Varese (Italy), Zaragova and Navarra (Spain), Geneva (Switzerland) and Calvados (France). Int J Cancer 1988; 41:483–91.

Wynder EL, Covey LS, Mabuchi K, Mushinski M. Environmental factors in cancer of the larynx: a second look. Cancer 1976; 38:1591–601.

Yokoyama A, Muramatsu T, Ohmori T, et al. Alcohol-related cancers and aldehyde dehydrogenase-2 in Japanese alcoholics. Carcinogenesis 1998; 19:1383–7.

Yu MC. Nasopharyngeal carcinoma: epidemiology and dietary factors. IARC Sci Publ 1991; 105:39–47.

2

Imaging head and neck cancer

David Salvage

Imaging modalities

The imaging modalities available for imaging head and neck cancer are ultrasound, CT, MRI, and PET-CT. Each has different advantages and disadvantages so the best modality for particular aspects of head and neck cancer evaluation should be used.

Ultrasound

Advantages

- High resolution
- Real time
- No ionising radiation
- Demonstrates internal architecture, pattern of vascular supply to cervical lymph nodes

Disadvantages

- Operator dependent
- Limited field of view
- Poor demonstration of primary tumors

CT

Advantages

- High resolution
- Quick acquisition (typically 10–15 seconds)
- Good demonstration of cortical bone involvement

Disadvantages
- Ionising radiation
- Relatively poor soft-tissue contrast
- Lymph node size, necrosis, extracapsular extension only

MRI

Advantages
- Good soft-tissue contrast
- Good demonstration of bone marrow involvement (**Figure 2.1**)
- Good demonstration of perineural/intracranial extension (**Figure 2.2**)

Disadvantages
- Moderate resolution
- Slow acquisition (typically 2.5–6.5 minutes per sequence, six sequences)
- Many safety issues (see the next section)

PET–CT

Advantages
- Demonstrates tissues with increased metabolic activity
- Can help distinguish post-treatment changes from recurrent disease

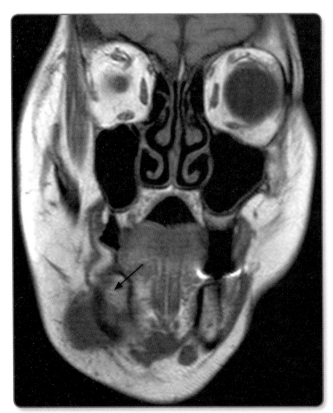

Figure 2.1 Coronal T1-weighted MRI showing direct tumor invasion through the cortex and into the marrow of the body of the mandible (black arrow).

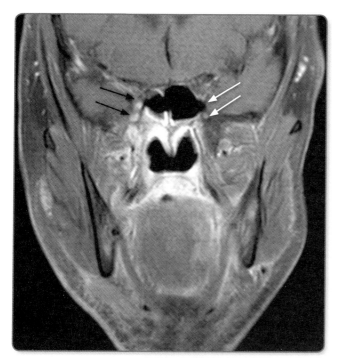

Figure 2.2 Coronal T1-weighted MRI with gadolinium enhancement and fat suppression demonstrating perineural extension of tumor. Enlargement and enhancement of the right maxillary division of the trigeminal nerve (superior) and nerve of the pterygoid canal (inferior) (black arrows) compared to the normal nerves on the left (white arrows).

- Covers whole body so can demonstrate distant metastatic disease (**Figure 2.3**)

Disadvantages
- Low resolution
- Slow acquisition, typically 30 minutes
- Ionising radiation

Safety issues

All imaging modalities have the potential to have harmful effects on human tissues and systems. Most are rare or minor, but occasionally significant harm can be caused. Awareness, and where possible prevention or mitigation, of such effects is vital for patient safety.

Ultrasound
- Potential heating of tissues (mainly early pregnancy)

CT

- Reactions to intravenous iodinated contrast media (American College of Radiologists (ACR) Committee on Drugs and Contrast Media 2012)
- Contrast-induced renal failure (ACR Committee on Drugs and Contrast Media 2012)
- Cumulative radiation dose from sequential scans (potentially)

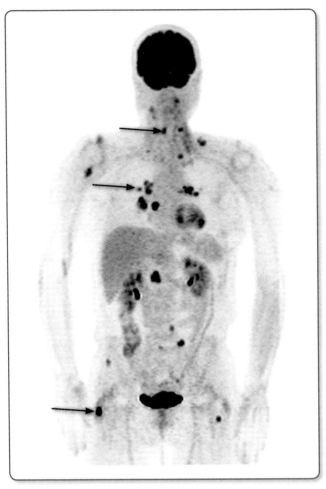

Figure 2.3 PET–CT scan of the whole body demonstrating locoregional and distant metastatic recurrence of previous oral cavity squamous cell carcinoma. Locoregional lymphadenopathy in the neck (top arrow), distant lymphadenopathy at the hila and distant metastases in the lungs (middle arrow) and distant metastases in the bones (bottom arrow).

MRI

Each MRI unit should have its local safety check list and there may be slight variations.

- Contraindications (absolute and relative)
  - Implanted stimulators, particularly cardiac pacemakers
  - Metal fragments in eyes/body (shrapnel, piercings)
  - Intracranial aneurysm clips
- Considerations
  - Artificial implants (e.g. joints, pins, plates, ears, eyes, and dental prostheses)
  - Heart surgery/valve replacement
  - Stents
  - Operation within preceding 6 weeks
  - Claustrophobia
- Reactions to intravenous gadolinium contrast media (ACR Committee on Drugs and Contrast Media 2012)

- Nephrogenic systemic fibrosis (ACR Committee on Drugs and Contrast Media 2012)

PET–CT

- Cumulative radiation dose from sequential scans (radioisotope and low-dose CT). Currently, the lowest dose for each scan is around 13 mSv, equivalent to 650 chest radiographs.

Staging the primary tumor

The preferred modality (CT or MRI) is partly dependent on availability of local resources and expertise (equipment and radiologists).

Generally, MRI is used for suprahyoid tumors of the nasal and oral cavities, nasopharynx, and oropharynx because there is limited movement of structures and good soft-tissue contrast. Contra-indications may make CT necessary instead.

CT is commonly used for infrahyoid tumors of the larynx and hypopharynx because there is greater potential for movement (swallowing), acquisition times are much shorter than MRI and the laryngeal skeleton is easier to appreciate.

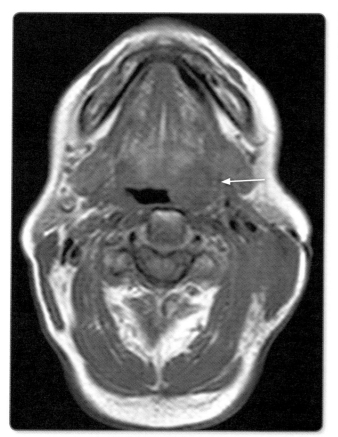

Figure 2.4 Transaxial T1-weighted MRI through the oropharynx showing a squamous cell carcinoma of the left tonsil (arrow).

Superficial mucosal tumors may be difficult to identify and their extent may be best appreciated on clinical examination.

Imaging technique

MRI

- At least two planes (axial and coronal)
- Skull base to thoracic inlet (axial)
- Tip of nose to cervical spinal canal (coronal)
- T1-weighted sequences (**Figure 2.4**)
- T2-weighted with fat suppression/STIR sequences (**Figure 2.5**)
- Gadolinium enhanced T1 sequences with fat suppression (**Figure 2.6**)

CT

- Intravenous iodinated contrast enhancement (100 mL 300 mg/mL I_2 at 1 mL/s)

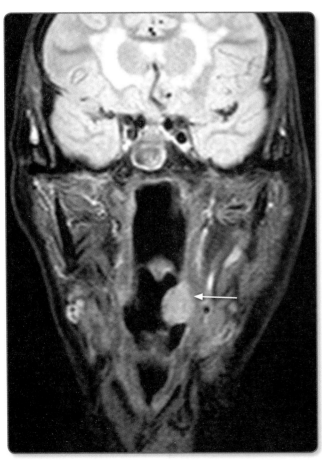

Figure 2.5 Coronal STIR MRI through the oropharynx showing a squamous cell carcinoma of the left tonsil (arrow).

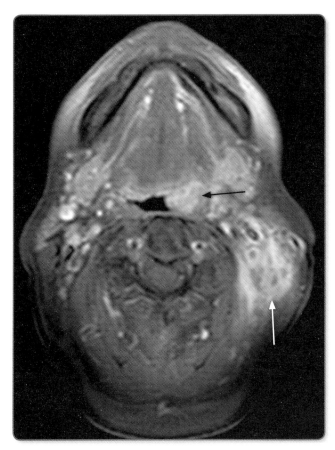

Figure 2.6 Transaxial T1-weighted MRI with gadolinium enhancement and fat suppression showing a squamous cell carcinoma of the left tonsil (black arrow). There is also ipsilateral level II lymphadenopathy with nodal extracapsular extension and invasion of the underlying and overlying muscles (white arrow).

- The patient swallows prior to the data acquisition to reduce the chance of swallowing during the scan
- Gentle respiration to prevent adduction of the vocal cords
- Axial acquisition from skull base to thoracic inlet with coronal (and sagittal) reformatted images (**Figure 2.7**)

Larynx

Stage T1 and T2 glottic tumors are difficult to distinguish on imaging as vocal cord mobility cannot be readily assessed and clinical assessment of vocal cord mobility is required. Tumor extension into the paralaryngeal fat is considered to represent stage T3 tumor as it is assumed that this will prevent vocal cord movement. Involvement of the laryngeal skeleton or extralaryngeal extension stages the tumor as T4.

Hypopharynx

Tumor staging is best determined clinically because tumors are often superficial or ulcerated making an assessment of their extent on imaging difficult. Deep extension/infiltration can be evaluated and if present upstages the tumor to T4.

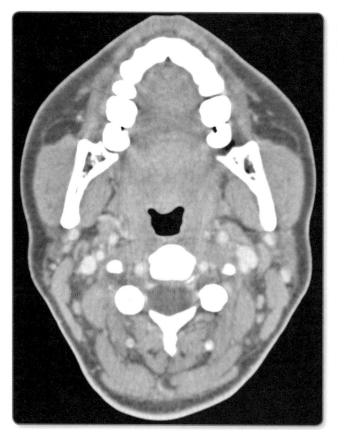

Figure 2.7 Transaxial CT scan with intravascular contrast enhancement through the oral cavity and oropharynx.

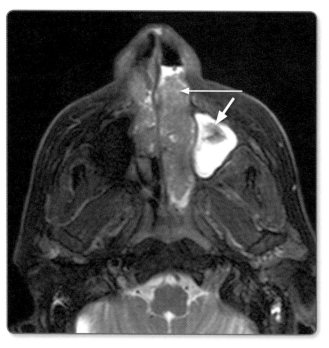

Figure 2.8 Transaxial T2-weighted MRI with fat suppression showing tumor of intermediate T2 signal in the nasal cavities (long, thin arrow) and obstruction of the left maxillary antrum with secondary inflammatory mucosal thickening and fluid of high T2 signal (short, thick arrow).

Sinonasal tumors

Soft tissue and bone information is required for staging and planning treatment which may include surgical reconstruction, so CT and MRI are required in most instances. CT demonstrates the extent of bone destruction and erosion of cortical bone. MRI distinguishes tumor from entrapped secretions and mucosal inflammation secondary to sinus obstruction (**Figure 2.8**), allowing more accurate demonstration of tumor extent.

Nasopharynx

Deep extension is difficult to assess clinically but MRI demonstrates this very well, particularly involvement of the bone marrow at the skull base, the parapharyngeal soft tissues and retropharyngeal lymphadenopathy.

CT may be complementary if partial erosion of cortical bone with small tumors needs to be excluded.

Oropharynx

The main role for imaging is to assess the deep and submucosal extension of tumor.

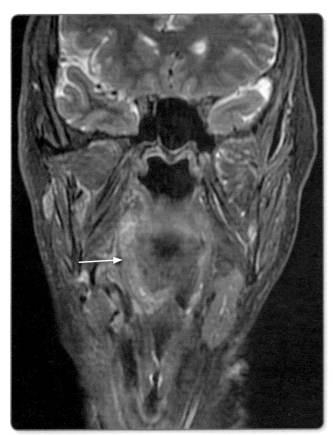

Figure 2.9 Coronal STIR MRI showing diffuse increased T2 signal in the right tonsillar bed extending from the soft palate to the vallecula 7 days after tonsillectomy. Small volume residual tumor cannot be distinguished from postoperative changes.

If possible, imaging should be performed before tonsillectomy as the early postoperative changes associated with this are often difficult to differentiate from small volume residual disease, particularly in the adjacent soft palate and tongue base (**Figure 2.9**).

Oral cavity

The extent of superficial tumors of the buccal mucosa can be difficult to demonstrate on imaging, and staging is best assessed clinically. The involvement of deeper tissues is well shown by imaging.

Occasionally, there can be significant clinically undetectable deep extension of tumors into the tongue, so MRI staging should be performed even if the tumor is superficially small (**Figure 2.10**).

Gingival/alveolar tumors can involve the bone marrow of the mandible or maxilla without eroding cortical bone, gaining access along the periodontal membrane, so MRI is the preferred method of imaging to evaluate this.

However, many patients with oral cancer have poor oral and dental hygiene and consequently poor dentition with caries and low-grade infection. This produces similar imaging appearances to tumor in the

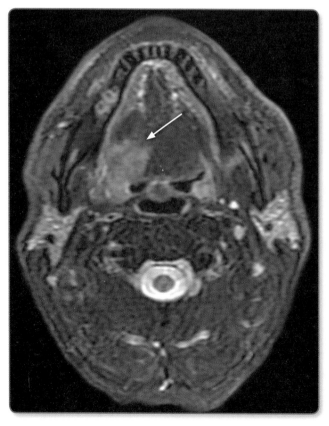

Figure 2.10 Transaxial T2-weighted MRI with fat suppression showing deep extension of a squamous cell carcinoma into the tongue (arrow). This was only apparent clinically as a small ulcer on the posterolateral right tongue base.

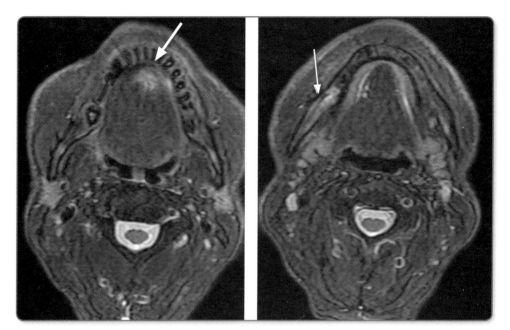

Figure 2.11 Transaxial T2-weighted MRI with fat suppression showing a small squamous cell carcinoma of the floor of the mouth (thick arrow) and inflammatory changes in the right mandible remote from the tumor and secondary to poor dental hygiene and dental infection (thin arrow).

bone marrow (**Figure 2.11**). If the changes are remote from the tumor then they can be reasonably ascribed to dental-related pathology. When the changes are adjacent to the tumor, tumor infiltration should be considered the most likely cause.

Staging neck disease

The neck should be included as part of the staging scan for the primary tumor.

The main features on CT or MRI that determine metastatic lymphadenopathy are lymph node size (>10 mm short transverse axis) and central non-enhancement indicating necrosis (**Figure 2.12**). The fatty hilum of the lymph node can mimic necrosis, but is usually eccentric and in continuity with the adjacent interstitial fat of the neck. (**Figure 2.13**).

Unequivocal metastatic lymphadenopathy demonstrated on the staging CT or MRI scan does not require further imaging of that side of the neck as it will be treated appropriately (usually neck dissection).

Further imaging of the neck lymph nodes with ultrasound should be considered:

- If the CT or MRI scan is equivocal for lymphadenopathy
- To assess the 'contralateral' side of the neck if no lymphadenopathy is demonstrated on this side on the CT or MRI staging scan,

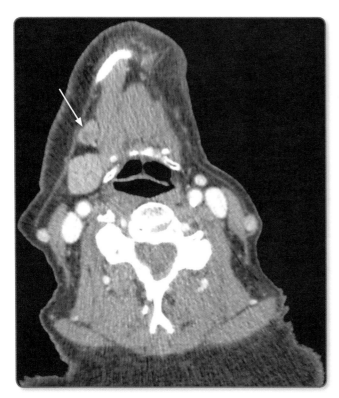

Figure 2.12 Transaxial CT scan with intravascular contrast enhancement showing a small right submandibular metastatic lymph node (arrow) from an ipsilateral oral cavity squamous cell carcinoma. The patchy reduced enhancement within the lymph node indicates necrosis.

particularly if the primary tumor extends across the midline or has a high propensity for metastatic spread to lymph nodes
- To guide fine needle aspiration cytology (FNAC) if confirmation of metastatic lymph node involvement is required

Staging distant metastases

Lungs

The most common site for distant metastases in head and neck cancers is the lungs, 66% of distant metastases (Ferlito et al. 2001).

Synchronous primary tumors of the lung are also found in 4–5% of patients with head and neck cancer, undoubtedly related to smoking as the common risk factor (Ghosh et al. 2009).

Chest radiograph

When the primary tumor is staged with an MRI, a chest radiograph may suffice to assess for a synchronous lung primary tumor when the likelihood for pulmonary metastases is low:
- Small primary tumor
- No cervical metastatic lymphadenopathy

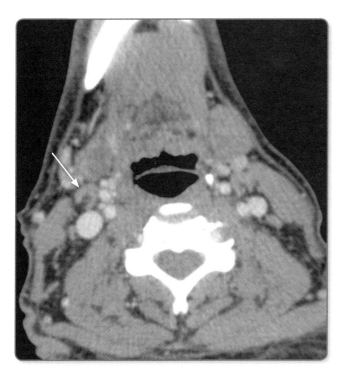

Figure 2.13 Transaxial CT scan with intravascular contrast enhancement showing a normal right level II lymph node (arrow). The low attenuation fatty hilum is in continuity with the adjacent interstitial fat.

CT chest

This is often performed when the primary tumor is staged with a CT scan.

It should always be performed when the primary tumor is staged with an MRI or CT and:

- Large primary tumor (T3+, occasionally large T2)
- Cervical metastatic lymphadenopathy N2+
- Vascular invasion on imaging

Liver

Reported in 10% but not routinely imaged (Ferlito et al. 2001):

- CT for demonstration
- MRI for characterization
- US to guide biopsy

Bone

Reported in 22% but not routinely imaged (Ferlito et al. 2001):

- Bone isotope scan if suspected clinically
- MRI for spine to differentiate metastases from degenerative disease

PET–CT

PET–CT is being increasingly used to assess the whole body for distant metastases when the patient has symptoms to suggest metastases or there is increased likelihood for these:

- Large primary tumor (T3+, occasionally large T2)
- Cervical metastatic lymphadenopathy N2+
- Vascular invasion on imaging

The low-spatial resolution makes the detection of metastases < 4 mm unlikely. This is compounded in the lungs and to a lesser extent in the liver by respiratory movement that causes any metastases to move during the acquisition of image data and to be 'blurred out.' Pulmonary metastases < 8 mm are difficult to demonstrate reliably.

Unknown (occult) primary tumors

Head and neck tumors often present as metastatic cervical lymphadenopathy. In many cases, a primary tumor can be identified on initial clinical examination.

When such a primary tumor is not evident, imaging complements upper aerodigestive tract endoscopy with biopsies and tonsillectomy in trying to identify the primary site. After such evaluation, < 5% primary head and neck cancers remain occult (Schwartz & Saltman 2012).

An MRI is preferred to CT scan because of the greater soft-tissue contrast between normal and abnormal tissues and reasonable spatial resolution.

PET–CT allows assessment for more distant primary tumors (e.g. lung) and distant metastatic spread, but has poor spatial resolution and may not demonstrate small primary tumors.

MRI and PET–CT are probably complementary and both should be performed if facilities exist.

If possible the imaging should be performed prior to 'surgical' endoscopy because:

- It may demonstrate a small tumor and direct more limited biopsies
- Both MRI and PET–CT will be abnormal at the site of tonsillectomy for at least 2 weeks after the operation and may be slightly abnormal at the other biopsy sites. This confounds imaging assessment for a possible head and neck primary tumor

However, the need for rapid investigation for and identification of a primary tumor often means that:

- Imaging is obtained after the 'surgical' endoscopy
- MRI and PET–CT should be requested at the same time rather than sequentially

Post-treatment imaging

Early postoperative period

Imaging during the early postoperative period is largely confined to the assessment of healing/integrity of the surgical closure after laryngectomy, prior to the recommencement of oral intake and commencement of adjuvant radiotherapy or chemoradiotherapy.

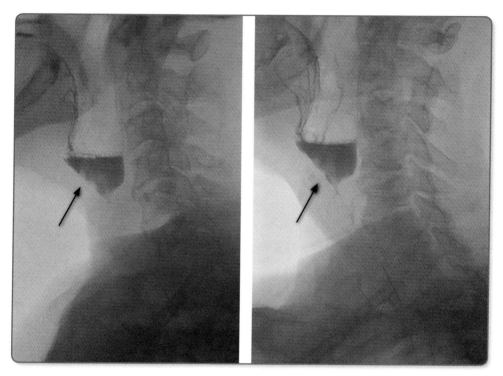

Figure 2.14 Lateral projections from a single contrast water-soluble swallow 10–14 days after laryngectomy. The image on the left from the first swallow of contrast shows a small collection of gas in the soft tissues anterior to the surgical closure of the hypopharynx but no leak of contrast. The image on the right from the fourth swallow of contrast shows a small amount of contrast within the gas collection indicating a minor delayed leak from the line of surgical closure.

A leak or fistula evident clinically does not require imaging.

A single-contrast swallow study using a water-soluble contrast medium is performed, ideally 10–14 days after the operation. A minimum of lateral and frontal projections and a repeated lateral projection at the end of the study are required to confirm healing and exclude a small 'delayed' leak at the suture line (**Figure 2.14**).

An obvious anastomotic leak on the initial (lateral) swallow does not require further projections at the time, but a repeat study after an appropriate period of time (1–2 weeks).

Post-treatment 'baseline' imaging

This should be performed at 3 months after completion of all treatment modalities (The Royal College of Radiologists 2006). Some of the early postoperative and acute post-treatment changes such as mucositis should have largely settled and much of the response to radiotherapy and chemotherapy will have become apparent.

The same imaging modality as the pretreatment staging scan should be used to make the assessment of treatment response easier.

Expected post-treatment changes

Postoperative
- Resected tumor and surrounding tissues
- Neck dissection(s)
- Flap reconstruction(s)

Radiotherapy related
- Tumor shrinkage (hopefully)
- 'Edema' around the tumor site
- 'Edema' in the irradiated fat, usually the subcutaneous and interstitial fat of the neck (may be unilateral) and within the larynx (epiglottis, aryepiglottic folds and false vocal cords)

Post-treatment 'follow-up' imaging

After the post-treatment 'baseline' imaging, planned follow-up scans are indicated if:
- The primary tumor site cannot be easily assessed clinically, e.g. difficult access to see directly, large flap reconstruction covering the tumor bed
- There is clinical/imaging concern for residual disease on the baseline scan

Imaging of treatment complications

Problems with swallowing
- Radiation-induced stricture – long, smooth
- Postoperative anastomotic stricture – short, smooth
- Hypertonic pharyngo-esophageal segment – after laryngectomy
- Recurrent tumor

Initial investigation with barium swallow

This will help differentiate normal post-treatment changes from recurrent disease (**Figure 2.15**). If recurrent disease demonstrated or suspected, CT scan to demonstrate extent and local spread (primary tumor likely to have been staged with CT scan rather than MRI so easier to compare, and the problems with swallowing require the shortest possible time for image acquisition)

Problems with voice production after surgical voice restoration
- 'Wet' voice
- Weak voice

Investigate with videofluoroscopy swallow in conjunction with speech and language therapist.

Osteoradionecrosis

It occurs after radiation treatment. Expected postradiation changes may make the interpretation of scans more difficult, but as osteoradionecrosis (ORN) is usually a delayed post-treatment complication, the postradiation changes on the post-treatment baseline scan have often resolved.

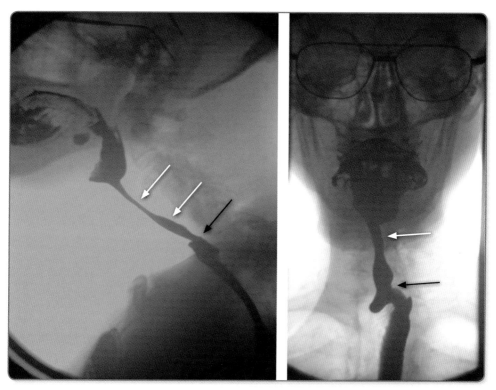

Figure 2.15 Lateral and frontal projections from a barium swallow several years after laryngectomy in a patient with worsening dysphagia. Smooth irregularity at the lower end of surgical closure (black arrow) is the postoperative anatomical configuration. Above this the smooth narrowing of the lower reconstructed hypopharynx (thick white arrow) is the result of surgical closure. The smooth greater narrowing of the upper reconstructed hypopharynx (thin white arrow) is an additional delayed postradiation stricture.

ORN can be difficult to differentiate from infection/osteomyelitis on imaging, as there are often soft-tissue changes adjacent to ORN as well as osteomyelitis.

A CT scan with intravenous contrast is the initial investigation to demonstrate the affected bones, particularly fragmentation of bone, destruction of bony trabeculae, and locules of gas within the bone (**Figure 2.16**). Associated soft-tissue changes can usually be appreciated but these can be further imaged with MRI if necessary.

Recurrent disease

Primary site

The preferred imaging modality is the same as the initial primary tumor staging unless there are patient incompatibilities, usually with MRI in which case a CT scan can be substituted.

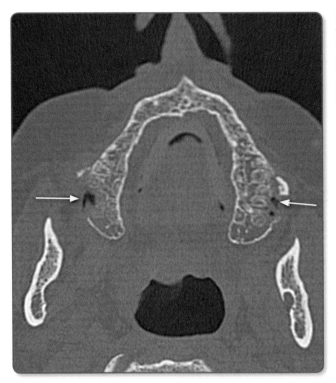

Figure 2.16 Transaxial CT scan through the oral cavity and oropharynx on bone windows showing osteoradionecrosis. There is fragmentation of and gas within the bone of the maxilla bilaterally (arrows).

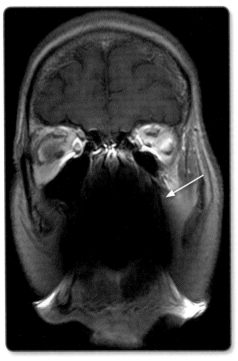

Figure 2.17 Coronal T1-weighted MRI with gadolinium enhancement showing the susceptibility effects of a dental prosthesis/obturator (black arrow). Distortion of adjacent anatomy and absent signal around and beyond the prosthesis obscures the oral cavity which is the region of interest in this instance (assessing for local recurrence of oral squamous cell carcinoma).

Intraoral obturators and facial bone reconstructions can produce considerable image distortion and loss of signal on MRI (**Figure 2.17**) and beam-hardening artefact on CT around the site of initial tumor resection, making it impossible to assess for small and moderate volume recurrent disease on imaging. In this situation, clinical assessment remains the only option, but MRI and/or CT should be tried once.

Neck

Recurrent disease/lumps presenting in the neck should be assessed initially with ultrasound to allow the nature of lymphadenopathy and other lumps to be determined, and to guide FNAC/biopsy.

If recurrent disease is confirmed in the neck:

- image primary site, to assess for recurrence (as above)
- CT scan of the chest to look for possible distant metastatic disease.

Distant

Recurrent disease presenting as distant metastases is not common from a head and neck primary tumor, and metastases from other primary tumors do occur in patients with previous head and neck cancer.

The search for another primary tumor should be performed:

- CT chest, abdomen and pelvis (together with MRI/CT of the head and neck cancer primary site)
  and/or
- PET-CT

Second primary tumors

Second primary tumors (Priante et al. 2011, Samant 2012) occur in up to 27% patients presenting with a clinically evident head and neck tumor. These can be:

- Synchronous and identified within 6 months of the initial presentation, or
- Metachronous and identified more than 6 months after the initial presentation

These tumors are usually in the head and neck, lung or esophagus.

Synchronous head and neck tumors

Careful and detailed scrutiny of the primary tumor staging and baseline follow-up scans for a possible second tumor separated by at least 2 cm from the initial identified tumor.

Synchronous lung tumors

See Section 'Staging distant metastases' – Subsection 'Lungs.'

If a synchronous lung tumor is identified, the staging and imaging investigations should be co-ordinated with the appropriate clinicians and multidisciplinary team (MDT).

Metachronous head and neck tumors

Patients usually present with another tumor at least 2 cm from the original tumor site or after 5 years if within 2 cm of the original tumor site.

Imaging investigation should be the same as for staging the initial primary tumor, neck and distant metastases (see Section 'Staging the primary tumor').

Metachronous lung tumors

Patients do not usually present to the head and neck cancer team and would be investigated and staged for a primary lung tumor by the appropriate clinicians and MDT.

Further reading

Ahuja A, Evans R (eds). Practical Head and Neck Ultrasound, vol. 4. London: Publishers Greenwich Medical Media Limited, 2000:67–83.

The Royal College of Radiologists. Recommendations for Cross-Sectional Imaging in Cancer Management: Computed Tomography – CT Magnetic Resonance Imaging – MRI Positron Emission Tomography - PET-CT. Issue 2. London. Royal College of Radiologists, 2006; Chapter 6 Head and neck cancers: 39-49.

References

ACR Committee on Drugs and Contrast Media. Adverse Events after Intravascular Iodinated Contrast Media Administration. ACR Manual on Contrast Media – Version 8. 2012; 6:21–8.

ACR Committee on Drugs and Contrast Media. Contrast-Induced Nephrotoxicity. ACR Manual on Contrast Media – Version 8. 2012; 8:33–41.

ACR Committee on Drugs and Contrast Media. Adverse Reactions to Gadolinium-Based Contrast Media. ACR Manual on Contrast Media – Version 8. 2012; 12:59–62.

ACR Committee on Drugs and Contrast Media. Nephrogenic Systemic Fibrosis (NSF). ACR Manual on Contrast Media – Version 8. 2012; 13:63–71.

Ahuja A, Evans R (eds). Practical Head and Neck Ultrasound, vol. 4. London: Publishers Greenwich Medical Media Limited, 2000:67–83.

Ferlito A, Shaha AR, Silver CE, et al. Incidence and sites of distant metastases from head and neck cancer. ORL J Otorhinolaryngol Relat Spec 2001; 63:202–7.

Ghosh SK, Roland NJ, Kumar A, et al. Detection of synchronous lung tumors in patients presenting with squamous cell carcinoma of the head and neck. Head Neck 2009; 31:1563–70.

Priante AV, Castilho EC, Kowalski LP. Second primary tumors in patients with head and neck cancer. Curr Oncol Rep 2011; 13:132–7.

Samant S. Second primary malignancies in patients with head and neck cancers. http://www.uptodate.com November 2012.

Schwartz DL, Saltman BE. Head and neck squamous cell carcinoma of unknown primary. http://www.uptodate.com. (Last accessed June 2012.)

The Royal College of Radiologists. Recommendations for Cross-Sectional Imaging in Cancer Management: Computed Tomography – CT Magnetic Resonance Imaging – MRI Positron Emission Tomography - PET-CT. Issue 2. London. Royal College of Radiologists, 2006; Chapter 6 Head and neck cancers: 39-49.

3

Therapy requirements in head and neck oncology

Ruth A. Simpson, Liz K. Wells and Elizabeth Nelson

Nutritional therapy

Head and neck cancer patients often present a challenge to health care professionals due to the multifactorial nature of their disease. As physical, medical, and social needs can alter throughout and after treatment, all health care professionals must be specialized and experienced in their field to respond appropriately (Ravasco et al. 2003). Malnutrition was identified as an adverse prognostic factor in head and neck cancer over 25 years ago (Brookes 1985), with , approximately 50–75% of patients identified as malnourished at diagnosis (van Bokhorst-de van der Schueren et al. 1997, Hammerlid et al. 1998), making it essential that the dietitian is a core member of the multidisciplinary team (MDT).

What is a dietician?

In the United Kingdom, all dietitians are required to be registered with the Health and Care Professions Council (HCPC). The title dietitian can only be used if the individual is appropriately trained and registered with the HCPC. They are statutorily-regulated and qualified to assess, diagnose and treat nutritional problems using scientific research and medical understanding, in both the acute hospital and community setting.

What is a head and neck dietician?

Head and neck cancer specialist dietitians are uniquely placed to follow patients from diagnosis, through surgery, postoperatively in the intensive care setting, through chemotherapy and radiotherapy treatment, to recovery and rehabilitation or end of life care. Dietitians play a key role in educating patients and carers on the nutritional impact of their treatment pathway and what to expect from artificial nutrition implementation. In the United Kingdom, the National Institute for Health and Care Excellence (NICE 2004) advise that head and neck cancer services should be centralized into specialist centers, with ongoing local support for rehabilitation and to ensure the continuation of care. A systematic review demonstrated that individualized dietary counseling by a dietitian had a more beneficial effect on nutritional status and quality of life in head and neck patients than no counseling and standard advice (Langius et al. 2013).

The key contributions of the dietitian to the MDT are as follows:

- Able to identify and anticipate patients who are nutritionally depleted or likely to become so
- Calculation of protein, energy, fluid and micronutrient requirements, based on age, gender, level of activity and clinical condition (Henry 2005)
- Expertise in complex nutritional support including artificial feeding and feeding tube selection
- Prescription of tailored nutrition support via oral, enteral or parenteral nutrition
- Advanced communication skills

Professor Marinos Elia defined malnutrition as 'a state of nutrition in which a deficiency or excess (or imbalance) of energy, protein and other nutrients causes measurable adverse effects on tissue/body form, body function and clinical outcome' (Thomas 2001). Numerically, malnutrition is defined as a weight loss of $> 10\%$ body weight over a 6 month period (van Bokhorst-de van der Schueren et al. 1997) or a body mass index (BMI) < 20 kg/m^2 at presentation if no weight loss is present. Early screening and dietary intervention are key as patients with a significant weight loss (10%) presurgery are at a higher incidence (20–50%) of postoperative complications (Bertrand et al. 2002).

Head and neck cancer has a profound effect on the nutritional status of its sufferers. To confound matters further many individuals present with a very poor nutritional status at diagnosis due to lifestyle choices such as alcoholism. The tumor mass often induces symptoms such as pain, discomfort, taste changes and obstruction on eating. Oral intake can become inadequate, restricted or impossible for prolonged periods of time prior to and during treatment due to temporary and/or permanent changes. To prevent and correct nutritional depletion, patients must be screened and receive timely intervention from the dietitian to overcome physical, social and psychological challenges.

Malnutrition has physiological and psychological consequences, impairing recovery, increasing length of stay and increasing costs to the National Health Service. Malnutrition and failure to meet a patient's significantly increased nutritional requirements may lead to complications such as infection, development of fistulae, and breakdown of anastomoses, poor wound healing and sepsis.

Causes of malnutrition in head and neck cancer patients, leading to many of these patients being at high-risk of refeeding syndrome (Thomas 2001, NICE 2006), include the following:

- Poor dietary habits
- Poor nutritional status prior to diagnosis
- Excessive alcohol intake, smoking, drug use
- Depression and anxiety
- Limited social network/familial support

- Homelessness
- Taste changes
- Difficulty with chewing and swallowing
- Cachexia

Nutritional effects of treatment

Head and neck cancer patients' nutritional requirements are high due to the patients' clinical condition and treatment interventions that can include radiotherapy, chemotherapy and major surgery. Increased requirements are required in order for a patient's optimum recovery, for example to ensure wound healing, prevent malnutrition, and aid rehabilitation. In addition to the factors that may cause malnutrition prior to diagnosis, the treatment itself can have a detrimental impact on a patient's nutritional status. Single or multimodality regimens (surgery, chemotherapy and radiotherapy) significantly increase the likelihood of nutritional depletion, immunosuppression and morbidity. Surgical resections can severely restrict or eliminate the ability to consume oral intake, therefore aggressive artificial nutrition support is imperative. A prospective randomized controlled trial in patients with head and neck cancer undergoing radiotherapy was carried out on 75 patients to determine the effect of dietary counseling and supplements on outcomes of nutrition and quality of life during and 3 months after radiotherapy. Over 90% of patients experienced radiotherapy toxicity. Researchers found that nutritional interventions and dietary counseling positively influenced outcomes. Nutritional intervention was a key to the improvements of patients nutritional and non-nutritional outcomes such as quality of life. Adding oral nutritional supplements to the diet did not seem to be as effective as dietary counseling (Ravasco et al. 2005).

The side effects of each treatment which cause side effects that impact on nutritional status can be seen in **Table 3.1**.

Nutritional requirements

The energy and protein requirements for an 80 kg man, aged 45 years, under different states of stress, are shown in **Table 3.2**. Basal metabolic rate (BMR) is calculated using Henry equations (Henry 2005). Additional activity levels must be added to BMR in addition to the stress of the condition. **Table 3.2** demonstrates the profound effect head and neck cancer treatment has on the body.

Increased nutritional requirements must be achieved through the use of dietary counseling and food fortification in the first instance. Once surgery has taken place or chemotherapy/radiotherapy is underway, achieving an individual's nutritional requirements becomes increasingly difficult. Oral nutritional supplements, enteral feeding via gastrostomy tubes or nasogastric tubes if appropriate, must be utilized. Only in circumstances where the gut has failed or is inaccessible should parenteral nutrition be used.

Table 3.1 Regimen side effects and their impact on nutritional status		
Treatment	Problem	Solution
Radiotherapy	Taste changes Distorted (metallic, sweet, salty, or 'cardboard') Abnormal and /or loss of taste.	Mouth care Avoid metal cutlery
	Mucositis: Pain Infection Retching 'Burning' sensation	Mouth care Appropriate food textures
	Fatigue Apathy and severe tiredness Daily travel for treatment Side effects of treatment Increased depressive state Reduced ability to prepare food if living alone	Increased support at home if possible
	Xerostomia (dry mouth): Temporary or permanent Causes difficulty with swallowing (patients can describe it as 'claggy' to eat food)	Requires good oral hygiene Artificial saliva spray may help Food texture modification (discuss with speech and language therapists) Additional fluids with meals, sauces, gravy, and sips of water can help
	Odynophagia (pain on swallowing): Caused by residual surgical problems Edema Xerostomia and mucositis Often can cause a decrease in appetite and food aversions	
	Dysphagia (swallowing difficulties): Pre-existing or as result of treatment Increased time and effort to consume meals leads to decreased intake Can result in unsafe swallow	Altered consistency of food (as recommended by speech and language therapists) Artificial feeding
	Trismus (restricted ability to open the mouth): Due to pre-existing tumor obstruction or radiotherapy induce Reduced intake	Modified texture Liquid diet
	Osteoradionecrosis: Permanent damage to mandible restricting ability to chew and resulting in trismus, pain difficulty eating and drinking	
	Wound healing: Permanent tissue damage and increased risk of wound breakdown, infection and necrosis.	
	Dental caries: Reduced/no saliva production can occur if treatment field includes parotid and submandibular glands	Ensure good oral hygiene

Contd...

Contd...

Treatment	Problem	Solution
Chemotherapy	Mucositis Although this may initially be radiotherapy induced, chemotherapy may exacerbate symptoms and reduce the capacity for healing	
	Diarrhea Distressing to patient Results in malabsorption of nutrition Can lead to dehydration	Ensure adequate fluid provision Alter osmolality of enteral feed
	Nausea and vomiting Systemic effect or anticipatory effect triggered by taste, smell and anxiety Will and desire to eat is reduced Changes in saliva quantity and consistency	
	Constipation Due to analgesic medication	Alter fiber and fluid content of feeds Ensure appropriate aperients are prescribed
Surgery	Loss of senses – taste and smell Reduced enjoyment of oral intake Reduce appetite Reduced enjoyment of mealtimes and a potential reduction in the social interaction of mealtimes	
	Difficulty in chewing, drooling, pocketing of food Increased effort and time to eat Reduction in intake due to embarrassment, withdrawal from social occasions/public eating	
	Chyle leak If untreated nutritional deficiencies will develop due to the loss of calories, protein and fat soluble vitamins Treatment consensus varies	If patient is able to feed orally utilize a very low fat diet, with added MCT supplementation to achieve nutritional needs If enteral feeding is possible use an MCT (medium chain triglyceride) feed If no enteral or oral feeding access can be gained, use parenteral nutrition.

Summary

Dietitians are uniquely positioned to ensure nutrition support is implemented in a timely and efficient manner via one-to-one nutritional counseling. Dietetic intervention ensures artificial feeding is correctly prescribed and malnutrition is directly addressed, resulting in a direct benefit on the physiological and psychological well-being of the patient, decreasing the potential for additional complications, potentially reducing the duration of the patient's length of stay and improving their quality of life through a grueling treatment process.

Table 3.2 Estimating nutritional requirements of adults taking into consideration metabolic effects of treatment (Todorovic & Micklewright 2011)

	Healthy individual	Chemotherapy/radiotherapy	Postoperative major surgery
Energy (kcal per day)	BMR = 1607 kcal	15–20% stress factor for chemo/radiotherapy = 1848–1928 kcal	25–40% stress factor for complex surgery = 2008–2249 kcal
Protein (g per day) (Elia 1990) Grams of $N_2 \times 6.25$ = protein in grams	0.17 g N_2/kg = 85 g	0.17–0.2 N_2/kg = 85–100 g protein	0.2–0.25 g N_2/kg = 100–125 g protein
Activity factor added to give final estimated requirement	PAL 1.5 = 2410 kcal	25% activity level assuming mobile around the ward or traveling for treatment = 2249–2329 kcal	15% sitting in bed = 2249–2490 kcal

BMR, basal metabolic rate.
Sedated and ventilated = 0%.
Bedbound and immobile = +10%.
Bedbound mobile/sitting = +15–20%.
Mobile on the ward = +25%.
Mobile in the community – utilize physical activity levels (PAL) based on occupational and non-occupational activity levels (Dietary reference values for food energy and nutrients for the United Kingdom 1991).
Other studies have provided a more concise method of calculating energy and protein requirements (Ravasco et al. 2005, Isenring et al. 2007).
When actual body weight is used in no non- obese mobile patients:
Energy ~ 30–35 kcal/kg per day.
Protein = 1.2 g/kg per day.

Speech and language therapy

What is a speech and language therapist (SLT)?

SLTs are trained to help children and adults who have difficulties with communication or with eating, drinking, and swallowing. They have expertise in assessing, diagnosing and managing a range of disorders, resulting in better health outcomes for their patients.

All SLTs working in the United Kingdom must be registered with the Health and Care Professions Council (HCPC) and meet their standards for training, professional skill, behavior, and health.

The Royal College of Speech and Language Therapists (RCSLT) is the professional body for speech and language therapy in the United Kingdom.

Communication

The term 'communication difficulty' is used to apply to any disorder of speech, language, or voice.

Eating, drinking and swallowing

The term 'eating, drinking, or swallowing difficulty' (commonly known as dysphagia) is used to refer to any disorder of the oral, pharyngeal, or esophageal stages of deglutition.

There are over 30 specific head and neck cancer sites and these encompass oral cancers (mouth, lip, and oral cavity), cancer of the larynx, cancer of the pharynx, thyroid cancer, and other relatively rare cancers such as salivary gland, nasal cavity, middle ear, and accessory sinus tumors (NICE 2004). SLTs work across the range of head and neck cancer sites, but predominantly with patients who present with tumors of the oral cavity, larynx, and pharynx.

Head and neck cancer – its impact on communication and swallowing

It is well known and documented that head and neck cancers can have devastating effects on the lives of patients; the treatment can be disfiguring and often makes normal speech and eating impossible (NICE 2004).

Treatment for most forms of head and neck cancer has permanent effects on organs essential for normal human activities like breathing, speaking, eating, and drinking (NICE 2004).

Speech and language therapy is therefore an integral part of the assessment and rehabilitation pathway for many head and neck cancer patients and the expertise of the therapist may be indicated at any point from prediagnosis through to palliative and end of life care.

The multi-disciplinary team (MDT) and speech and language therapy

The concept of MDT management is well established in head and neck cancer care. The SLT is a core member of this team, using a range of skills in communication and swallowing therapy to benefit the patient throughout the course of treatment intervention (NICE 2004).

The SLT is a core member of the head and neck multidisciplinary oncology team from the time of patient presentation (RCSLT 2005). They work within the MDT to consider the impact and possible consequences of a communication and/or swallowing disorder. The therapist can influence decision-making regarding treatment planning and the consequences for rehabilitation of speech, voice and swallowing.

Indeed, The British Association of Head and Neck Oncologists recommend that 100% of centers/units should have a named SLT with at least 50% of their time dedicated to head and neck cancer work and with specialist surgical voice restoration (SVR) skills (BAHNO 2009).

Further supporting evidence specifies that while the responsibility for the rehabilitation of voice, speech and swallowing rests with the whole MDT, it is the specific role of the SLT within the team to oversee it (BAOHNS 2011).

Key points of speech and language therapy involvement in the pathway

Patients will ideally be seen for assessment as soon as possible after diagnosis and before treatment commences (RCSLT 2005), but intervention may be indicated at any of the following stages in the pathway:

- Prediagnosis
- Diagnosis and care planning
- Treatment
- Post-treatment
- Monitoring and survivorship
- Palliative care
- End of life

Aspects of the role of the SLT

- To develop and support the communication skills of both the patient and communicative partners
- To have a unique role to play in a laryngeal voice restoration postlaryngectomy
- To have the lead responsibility for the decision-making process of prosthesis selection, care and management in SVR postlaryngectomy
- To contribute to better health outcomes through their unique role in assessing, diagnosing and managing patients who have an oropharyngeal dysphagia at both pre- and post-treatment stages. They are involved with MDT decision-making including the need for alternative/supplementary non-oral feeding
- To review objective measures, such as videofluoroscopy (VFS) and/or fiberoptic endoscopic evaluation of swallowing (FEES), to more thoroughly assess, diagnose and manage swallowing difficulties
- To monitor and review a patient's progress with swallowing over time in order to effectively manage any risk associated with the presence of transient, intermittent or persistent dysphagia
- To contribute to palliative and end-of-life care, maximizing and facilitating communication and managing dysphagia in order to improve quality of life where possible

Clinical evaluation of communication

A clinical evaluation of communication routinely consists of a comprehensive case history followed by consideration of the following specific aspects of assessment:

- Cognitive status
- Orofacial/cranial nerve examination
- Speech intelligibility
- Vocal function
- Literacy skills
- Preferred communication/language (interpreter may be required)
- Hearing
- Visual acuity
- Manual dexterity
- Psychosocial status, including occupation
- Concerns and expectations
- Current medication

Evaluation of these parameters enables the SLT to plan the most appropriate method for communication rehabilitation and to identify any augmentative or alternative methods of communication that may benefit the patient, e.g. mouthing, writing, gesture, the use of picture/letter/word-based charts, or electronic/computerized aids.

The SLT may discuss onward referral to other agencies if specific issues have been identified during the course of assessment, e.g. referral for psychological support.

Communication and the total laryngectomy

All patients undergoing total laryngectomy should be assessed by the SLT before surgery in order to determine the method of communication best suited to the individual. The options are as follows:

- Prosthetic SVR
- Electrolarynx (placed on the cheek/neck or by using an oral adapter)
- Esophageal voice
- Communication aids, e.g. low or high tech
- Mouthing, writing, drawing, or gesture

It is important to offer the patient the opportunity to meet a well adjusted total laryngectomy who has established a successful means of communication. Patients should also be made aware of recommended support agencies who produce high-quality and helpful literature.

Prosthetic SVR

Prosthetic SVR is a recognized procedure for postlaryngectomy voice rehabilitation. This procedure involves placing a medical grade silicone voice prosthesis into a surgically created tract within the tracheoesophageal party wall. Pulmonary air is redirected into the esophagus when the tracheostoma is covered and this airstream provides the energy source for vibration of the pharyngoesophageal (PE) segment of the upper digestive tract, so producing a 'pseudo' voice (Evans et al. 2010).

All patients should be assessed with a view to their suitability for primary SVR. Full discussion is required with the patient and their carers to ensure understanding of their responsibility for voice prosthesis maintenance and care and the need to seek prompt advice when needed. There are a number of contra-indications that preclude successful SVR and these are as follows:

- Poor cognition/dementia
- Limited oral movement
- Profound deafness/patient using sign language
- Poor vision with no carer support
- Limited manual dexterity with no carer support
- Patient refusal

Patients who undergo SVR will be seen by the SLT once clearance has been given by the surgical team to commence voice rehabilitation. The SLT will initiate the following:

- Provide a full explanation and obtain consent prior to the procedure
- Accurately size the tracheoesophageal puncture (TOP)

- Select and fit an appropriate voice prosthesis, minimizing discomfort and risk
- Demonstrate appropriate care and maintenance of the voice prosthesis
- Provide advice on voicing technique
- Down-size the voice prosthesis when indicated
- Provide advice on emergency procedures in the event of extrusion
- Provide advice on recognition and management of leakage
- In conjunction with ENT colleagues provide advice on management of candidal valve infestation
- Seek an ENT opinion promptly when complications are suspected
- Provide written information regarding emergency aid out of SLT working hours
- Accurately document and record information at each prosthesis change
- Carry out all procedures in line with local guidance and policy

Artificial larynx (electrolarynx)

An artificial larynx (electrolarynx) is a device that produces a sound to substitute that of the normal voice. It is commonly powered by rechargeable batteries and can usually be programmed for each individual in terms of pitch level and volume. It may be placed against the neck or cheek and the sound created can be modified by the resonatory and articulatory structures to produce speech. An oral adapter may be used in cases of ongoing wound healing, discomfort or swelling of the neck. Guidance and practice are needed to optimize use of these devices and to communicate in a way that is not distracting to the listener.

Esophageal voice

Esophageal voice involves the production of a 'voice' within the esophagus, using air swallowed by the individual. Air is expelled through a constriction in the esophagus formed by the cricopharyngeus muscle. When this narrowed segment (pharyngoesophageal or PE segment) vibrates, sound is produced (Casper & Colton 1998).

Advantages to this form of communication are that both hands are free during speech and the patient is independent of devices that may be visually distracting or need high levels of care and maintenance. Disadvantages are that esophageal voice may be difficult to master and may never be functional, particularly in cases of extensive surgery and where there are significant medical complications. Esophageal voice is more acceptable to the male than to the female patient.

Assessment for heat moisture exchanger systems

All patients who have undergone total laryngectomy should be assessed for a suitable filter system to ensure optimum pulmonary function due to the loss of the warming, moistening, filtering and resistance functions of the nose. These systems may be:

- Open humidification systems, e.g. foam or bib covers
- Closed humidification systems, e.g. stud, tube, or base-plate with a removable filter that can be disposed of and replaced
  Factors to consider in the selection of an appropriate system are as follows:
- Contour of the stoma
- Width and depth of the stoma
- Stoma patency
- Stoma sensitivity
- Skin integrity
- Manual dexterity
- Life-style
- Cosmetic appearance
- Patient preference

The properties and long-term benefits of closed humidification systems are far greater than open systems. Patients should be encouraged to trial various systems to determine the one that best fits their life-style and needs and affords the greatest protection. Many products are now available on prescription.

Assessment for hands-free speech

Many patients who have undergone total laryngectomy may wish to pursue hands-free speech. Hands-free speech refers to the use of an attachment inserted into the stoma stud, tube, or base-plate that removes the need to occlude the stoma with a finger or thumb for voicing. The SLT may carry out a pressure assessment to determine a patient's pressure range when voicing on sounds, single words and in connected speech. An ideal pressure range lies between 25 and 40 cm H_2O. Generation of high pressure when voicing will dislodge the stud/tube or loosen the base-plate creating air leakage. Conversely, generation of a low pressure range may fail to close the hands-free valve and voicing will not be possible.

Clinical evaluation of swallowing

A clinical evaluation of swallowing routinely consists of taking a comprehensive case history followed by consideration of the specific aspects of assessment listed:
- Level of alertness
- Emotional state, mood, and behavior
- Cognitive levels
- General motor skills and positioning
- Respiratory status/presence and type of tracheostomy tube
- Oral hygiene and dental health
- Management of secretions
- Oro-facial/cranial nerve examination
- Vocal tract function
- Nutrition, hydration, and dietary preferences
- Presence of gastroesophageal reflux
- Medication

Evaluation of the parameters listed enables the SLT to undertake a risk assessment in relation to current eating and drinking, determine the impact of the disorder and prioritize further assessment (RCSLT 2005).

Trials of fluid and food consistencies may be carried out using observational skill and practical application of laryngeal palpation to determine swallow safety and efficiency. Cervical auscultation and pulse oximetry may provide additional information to inform clinical decisions, but should not form the sole basis of clinical judgment. The following points should be considered when assessing fluid and food textures (RCSLT 2005):

- Fluid viscosity
- Food texture
- Bolus size
- Bolus placement
- Temperature
- Taste
- Pacing
- Adapted cups/modified utensils
- Intraoral prosthetics

Compensatory strategies

Compensatory strategies may be used to alter aspects of swallowing physiology, improve swallow function and reduce/eliminate laryngeal penetration/aspiration (Logemann 1998). These strategies are postural changes and swallow maneuvers.

Postural changes that may be used are as follows:

- Chin down
- Head tilt (to the stronger side)
- Head turn (to the damaged side)
- Head back
- Side lying

Swallow maneuvers that may be used are as follows:

- Effortful swallow (to improve posterior movement of the tongue base)
- Supraglottic swallow (to close the vocal folds before and during the swallow)
- Super-supraglottic swallow (to improve closure of the airway entrance)
- Mendelsohn maneuver (to increase extent and duration of laryngeal elevation)

Texture modification of food and fluid

In 2012, a system of national descriptors was developed by the National Patient Safety Agency (NPSA) in order to standardize food textures for dysphagic patients. The Dysphagia Diet Food Texture Descriptors are listed as follows:

- Thin puree dysphagia diet (Texture B)
- Thick puree dysphagia diet (Texture C)

- Premashed dysphagia diet (Texture D)
- Fork mashable dysphagia diet (Texture E)
  Fluid consistencies are generally classified as:
- Normal fluid
- Stage 1 (syrup) – pours quickly off a spoon
- Stage 2 (custard) – pours slowly off a spoon
- Stage 3 (pudding) – drips rather than pours off a spoon

At the conclusion of a clinical evaluation of swallowing, recommendations should be made for the safe and efficient delivery of fluid and food consistencies as appropriate. Close liaison is required with the dietitian, nursing, and catering staff to ensure that the patient receives adequate hydration and nutrition in a safe manner. Range of motion exercises may be provided to maintain or improve oromotor function for swallowing safety and efficiency.

As some components of the swallow cannot be accurately assessed clinically, there may be a need for instrumental evaluation. Two commonly used objective assessments are VFS and FEES. The choice of instrumental assessment should be guided by clinical indications, rather than by available resources and should always be preceded by a clinical swallowing evaluation.

Videofluoroscopic evaluation of oropharyngeal swallowing disorders

VFS is a modification of the standard barium swallow X-ray examination and is a hypothesis-driven adjunct to a full case history and clinical assessment of the patient. During a VFS, oropharyngeal swallowing anatomy and physiology is evaluated while the patient eats and drinks and the moving images are recorded for interpretation. Image recording enables the evaluation to be reviewed and shared with the patient, carer, and members of the MDT (RCSLT 2013).

The SLT must discuss the referral for VFS with the medical practitioner and patient, obtaining their consent in accordance with local guidelines. It is important that patients are appropriately selected for this procedure, with due consideration being given to the following contraindications:

- Medical instability
- Limited level of alertness
- Difficulty maintaining an appropriate position
- Poor co-operation
- Extreme distress
- Known or suspected adverse reaction to contrast media
- Portable ventilation not possible
- Patient pregnancy
- Nil By mouth for reasons other than dysphagia

VFS may assess in the lateral or anteroposterior planes and during the course of the study, positioning, swallow maneuvers and texture modifications to food or fluids may be trialed. At the conclusion of the assessment, oropharyngeal swallow features are analyzed with recommendations for optimizing swallow efficiency and safety.

SLTs have a unique role in the assessment and management of oropharyngeal dysphagia and play a key part in delivering VFS services within a multidisciplinary context. SLTs must have approval from their employer to undertake VFS and clinical competence must be evidenced by specialist training at a postgraduate level.

It is important to realize that a VFS provides a snapshot of a patient's swallow and, consequently, may not be wholly representative of their normal pattern of swallowing. The findings should therefore be applied within the context of the full case history and clinical observations.

Fiberoptic endoscopic evaluation of swallowing

FEES is an endoscopic examination of the pharyngeal stage of swallowing. It incorporates assessment of laryngopharyngeal anatomy and physiology as it relates to swallowing, assessment of swallowing function (saliva, fluid and food) and intervention to determine the postural and behavioral strategies that facilitate safer and more efficient swallowing (Kelly et al. 2007).

The SLT must discuss the referral for FEES with the medical practitioner and patient. It is important that patients are appropriately selected for this procedure, with due consideration being given to the following contraindications:

- Severe movement disorders and/or severe agitation
- Base of skull/facial fracture
- Recent history of severe/life-threatening epistaxis
- Sinonasal and anterior skull base tumors/surgery
- Nasopharyngeal stenosis

FEES may evaluate anatomy and swallow physiology; secretion management and sensation; airway protection as it relates to swallowing function; swallowing of foods/fluids; postures, strategies, and maneuvers; optimum delivery of bolus consistencies and sizes and therapeutic techniques.

FEES should be performed as a part of a MDT approach to dysphagia management.

Evaluation of SLT service provision

SLTs carry a responsibility to evaluate service provision to head and neck cancer patients. This may be carried out by:

- Use of service-specific outcome measures
- Service-based audit/research
- Contribution to the National Clinical Audit, e.g. data for head and neck oncology
- Contribution to the peer review process

MDT collaboration in SLT referral

Prompt and timely SLT referral from members of the MDT is valued in order to implement appropriate interventions. Examples of patients requiring prompt referral to the SLT are as follows:

- Patients who are unable to swallow or have difficulty swallowing and are judged to have an aspiration risk on fluid and/or food textures

- Patients due to undergo surgery for upper aerodigestive tract (UAT) tumors where communication/swallowing problems are a foreseeable consequence
- Patients due to undergo a course of radical radiotherapy or chemo-radiotherapy for UAT tumors
- Patients who have dysphagia on pureed diet and thickened fluids
- Patients planned for partial/total laryngectomy
- Patients planned for laser resection of the vocal cords (especially where significant resection is anticipated)
- Patients requiring pretreatment exercises
- Voice prosthesis leakage
- Extruded voice prosthesis (no stent in the puncture site)
- Problematic puncture/ill-fitting voice prosthesis
- Stoma management issues
- Patients wishing to meet an appropriately selected patient for support
  Some examples of situations where patients require routine SLT input are as follows:
- Heat moisture exchanger or filter assessment
- Hands-free speech assessment
- Routine voice prosthesis changes
- Voice prosthesis self-changing program
- Patient listed for secondary puncture
- Communication aid assessment, e.g. high- or low-tech aids
- Esophageal voice training
- Voice care and therapy
- Maximizing articulation/speech intelligibility
- Oromotor therapy (exercises to improve range, rate and strength of movement)

Further reading

Enderby P, Pickstone C, John A, et al. Resource Manual for Commissioning and Planning Services for SLCN (Head and Neck Cancer). RCSLT, 2009.

National Collaborating Centre for Acute Care. Nutrition Support in Adults Oral Nutrition Support, Enteral Tube Feeding and Parenteral Nutrition. London: National Collaborating Centre for Acute Care, 2006.

National Cancer Action Team (NCAT). Supporting and Improving Commissioning of Cancer Rehabilitation Services. Guidelines. London: NHS NCAT (archived material), 2009.

National Cancer Action Team (NCAT). Cancer Rehabilitation Pathway (Head and Neck) and Symptom Specific Pathways (Communication and Dysphagia). London: NHS NCAT (archived material), 2009.

Shaw C. Nutrition and Cancer. Oxford: Blackwell Publishing Ltd, 2011:188–220.

References

British Association of Head and Neck Oncologists (BAHNO). BAHNO Standards. London: British Association of Head and Neck Oncologists, 2009.

British Association of Otorhinolaryngologists Head and Neck Surgeons (BAOHNS). Head and Neck Cancer: Multidisciplinary Management Guidelines, 4th edn. London: Royal College of Surgeons, 2011.

Bertrand PC, Piquetm A, Bordier I, Monnier P, Roulet M. Preoperative nutritional support at home in

Head and neck cancer patients: from nutritional benefits to the prevention of the alcohol withdrawal syndrome. Curr Opin Clin Nutr Metab Care 2002; 5:435–40.

Brookes GB. Nutritional status – a prognostic indicator in head and neck cancer. Otolaryngol Head Neck Surg 1985; 93:69–74.

Casper JK, Colton RH. Clinical Manual for Laryngectomy and Head/Neck Cancer Rehabilitation, 2nd Revised Edition. San Diego, CA: Singular Publishing Group,1998.

Dietary reference values for food energy and nutrients for the United Kingdom. Report of the Panel on Dietary Reference Values of the Committee on Medical Aspects of Food Policy. Rep Health Soc Subj (Lond) 1991; 41:1–210.

Evans E, Hurren A, Govender R, et al. Prosthetic Surgical Voice Restoration (SVR): The Role of the Speech and Language Therapist. RCSLT Policy Statement. RCSLT, 2010.

Hammerlid E, Wirblad B, Sandin C, et al. Malnutrition and food intake in relation to quality of life in head and neck cancer patients. Head Neck1998; 20:540–8.

Henry CJ, Basal metabolic rate studies in humans: measurement and development of new equations. Public Health Nutr 2005; 8:1133–52.

Isenring EA, Bauer JD, Capra S. Nutrition support using the American Dietetic Association medical nutrition therapy protocol for radiation oncology patients improves dietary intake compared with standard practice. J Am Dietetic Assoc 2007;107:404–12.

Kelly AM, Hydes K, McLaughlin C, Wallace S. Fibreoptic endoscopic evaluation of swallowing (FEES): the role of speech and language therapy. RCSLT Policy Statement. RCSLT, 2007.

Langius JAE, Zandbergen MC, Eerenstein SEJ, et al. Effect of nutritional interventions on nutritional status, quality of life and mortality in patients with Head and neck cancer receiving (chemo) radiotherapy: a systematic review. Clin Nutr 2013; 32:671–8.

Logemann JA. Evaluation and Treatment of Swallowing Disorders, 2nd edn. Pro-Ed, Inc, 1998.

NICE. Improving Outcomes in Head and Neck Cancers – The Manual. London: National Institute for Clinical Excellence, 2004.

NPSA. Dysphagia diet food texture descriptors NPSA dysphagia expert reference group, 2012.

Ravasco P, Monteiro-Grillo I, Marques Vidal P, Camilo ME. Impact of nutrition on outcome: a prospective randomized controlled trial in patients with head and neck cancer undergoing radiotherapy. Head Neck 2005; 27:659–68.

Ravasco P, Monteiro-Grillo I, Vidal PM, Camilo ME. Nutritional deterioration in cancer: the role of disease and diet. Clin Oncol 2003; 15:443–50.

Royal College of Speech and Language Therapists. Videofluoroscopic evaluation of oropharyngeal swallowing function (VFS): The role of speech and language therapists. RCSLT Position Paper 2013. London: RCSLT, 2013.

Taylor-Goh S (ed). Royal College of Speech and Language Therapists; Department of Health (UK); National Institute for Clinical Excellence (NICE). RCSLT Clinical Guidelines: 5.8 Disorders of Feeding, Eating, Drinking & Swallowing (Dysphagia). RCSLT Clinical Guidelines. Bicester: Speechmark Publishing Ltd, 2005.

Thomas B, Bishops J. Manual of Dietetic Practice, 4th edn. Oxford: Blackwell Publishing Ltd, 2001:80–90, 769–79.

van Bokhorst DE, van der Schueren MA, van Leeuwen PA, et al. Assessment of malnutrition parameters in head and neck cancer and their relation to postoperative complications. Head Neck 1997; 19:419–25.

4 Systemic therapy in head and neck cancer

Angela Waweru and Martin H. Robinson

The basic principle of systemic therapy is DNA damage, either directly or indirectly leading to cell death.

Although the mainstay of non-surgical management in head and neck malignancies is radiotherapy, concurrent systemic therapy has a definite role, and has been shown to improve overall survival as well as progression free survival. In patients with incurable and/or metastatic disease, response to chemotherapy – even partial – can have a dramatic improvement in patients' symptoms and quality of life.

As will be discussed later, there are four main areas where systemic therapy is employed in the treatment of head and neck malignancies. Here, we discuss the main chemotherapeutic agents currently in use, common and serious side effects as well as the management of these.

Platinum agents: cisplatin and carboplatin

Platinum agents are among the most widely used chemotherapeutic agents. For many years, cisplatin was the only platinum agent available; however, analogs have been developed in a bid to reduce toxicity while maintaining efficacy.

Cisplatin's main mechanism of action is by binding to DNA causing adducts, the most lethal being intrastrand adducts that impair DNA replication and repair as well as inducing apoptosis. It is administered intravenously, over 1–2 hours; side effects include renal toxicity, nausea and vomiting, peripheral neuropathy, ototoxicity (tinnitus and deafness), infertility, and myelosuppression.

Prevention of cisplatin renal toxicity is achieved by ensuring an adequate baseline glomerular filtration rate (GFR) (>50 mL/min), hyperhydration prechemotherapy and being mindful of concomitant use of other nephrotoxic agents. Urine output is monitored during administration. Cisplatin is highly emetogenic. Management of nausea and vomiting has, however, improved with the advent of 5-HT$_3$ antagonists, e.g. ondansetron, used in combination with dexamethasone. Persistent or worsening ototoxicity requires reduction in the dose of cisplatin and if this does not improve symptoms, consideration should be made to stopping the drug otherwise patients are at risk of developing permanent tinnitus and hearing loss.

Carboplatin is an analog to cisplatin, it is a much more stable compound with a similar mode of action as cisplatin; it has less toxicities as there is a slower rate of DNA adduct formation and has comparable or less efficacy compared to cisplatin. It is eliminated as an intact molecule and its dose is therefore based on renal function [Calvert formula: Dose = AUC + (GFR + 25)].

It has more hematological toxicities compared to cisplatin with higher rates of myelosuppression recorded – thrombocytopenia is usually dose limiting. Emesis, nephrotoxicity, and neurotoxicity are uncommon. Other rare side effects include rash and anaphylaxis. Carboplatin can be substituted for cisplatin in patients with poor renal function in the palliative setting.

5-Fluorouracil (5FU)

5FU is an antimetabolite; these are drugs that interfere with DNA synthesis and therefore cell replication. It is an inactive compound that goes through complex metabolic activation. It is usually administered intravenously, although oral prodrugs now exist, e.g. capecitabine, that are preferentially activated in tumor cells.

In head and neck carcinoma treatment, 5FU is used in combination with cisplatin as their different modes of intracellular action lead to higher rates of cell kill; it is given as an infusion over 4 days as opposed to bolus administration; the main toxicities with this mode of administration are related to mucus membranes – e.g. mucositis; rare side effects include cardio toxicity (arrhythmias, coronary spasms), ataxia, and skin rash. Myelosuppression with infusional 5FU is uncommon.

Taxanes

These are agents that inhibit micro tubular disassembly. This prevents normal growth and differentiation of microtubules that are required for cell replication.

Docetaxel is the main agent used in head and neck cancer treatment typically as part of induction chemotherapy; it is excreted by hepatic metabolism via the cytochrome p450 system and therefore patients on drugs that affect this system (e.g. antiepileptic drugs) have altered docetaxel metabolism.

The main toxicities are myelosuppression (mainly neutropenia), hypersensitivity reactions, sensory peripheral neuropathy, fluid retention, and skin and nail changes.

Targeted biological agents

Targeted therapies are set to overtake the use of conventional chemotherapy in many disease sites. Certainly, in the context of head and neck malignancies, epidermal growth factor receptor (EGFR) inhibition has been shown to act synergistically with radiotherapy and improves overall survival when compared to radiotherapy alone.

The role of these agents is evolving and is discussed briefly toward the end of this chapter.

Acute oncology - management of toxicities

Bleeding and bruising

Thrombocytopenia due to chemotherapy-related myelosuppression e.g. carboplatin, (or occasionally disease-related marrow infiltration) should be managed according to approved guidelines. A platelet count of <50 can result in bleeding and or bruising from minor trauma. Higher incidences of intracranial hemorrhage have been recorded when there is sepsis plus a platelet count of <10. Typical management would include the following:

- Stop any drugs that could exacerbate bleeding such as antiplatelet therapy, warfarin or low molecular weight heparin
- In a stable patient with a platelet count of 10 or less, 1 unit of platelets should be administered
- Patients with sepsis and a count of <20 should have 1 unit of platelets administered
- Patients with evidence of bleeding in association with thrombocytopenia (platelets <50) should receive 1 unit of platelets

Diarrhea

Diarrhea can be a life-threatening complication of systemic therapies such as 5FU or cetuximab. If left untreated, prolonged or severe diarrhea can lead to acute kidney injury and hypovolemic shock. All patients with moderate or severe symptoms should be monitored closely, this includes, stool chart, fluid balance records, daily U&Es and abdominal examination to check for signs of peritonism. Stool micobiology and culture (MC&S) should be obtained to check for the possibility of an infective component:

- Mild to moderate diarrhea (increase by 2–3 or 4–6 bowel movements respectively) can be managed by stopping anticancer therapy after discussing with the appropriate team; stop any laxatives; loperamide on a PRN basis up to 16 mg/24 h plus codeine phosphate 30–60 mg PRN 4–6 hourly.
- Severe diarrhea (increase of >7 bowel movements): manage as above, and admit the patient for IV rehydration; consider adding octreotide. Buscopan can be administered via a syringe driver for diarrhea-related abdominal cramps (80 mg/24 h)

Mucositis

Typically seen with anti-metabolite drugs such as 5FU. Oral mucositis is commonly mistaken for candidiasis. (Any evidence of candidiasis should be treated with fluconazole syrup 50 mg o.d. for 7 days.) Patients with mucositis complain of sore mouth with sticky saliva. As higher rates of mucositis are seen in neutropenic patients, management in the first instance should be to exclude neutropenia; typical management of mucositis:

- Mouth care with combination of alcohol free mouthwash such as Biotene and Difflam mouthwash used pre-meals. Avoid chlorhexidine mouthwash
- Oxcetacaine and antacid taken half an hour before main meals can help with pain management. If swallowing is difficult, Mucilage 10 mL can used as an adjunct just prior to meals
- Systemic analgesia is gradually titrated up until effective pain control is reached, starting from regular soluble paracetamol 1 g QDS up to regular opiates if indicated. Care should be taken to avoid Oramorph solution due to its high alcohol content; morphine hydrochloride is preferable
- In severe cases, inpatient management is required for rehydration and dietetic support that could include parenteral nutrition (NG or TPN). Ongoing systemic therapy should always be stopped in these instances

Nausea and vomiting

Nausea and vomiting related to chemotherapy can be acute (<24 h) or delayed (2–5 days). Certain agents such as cisplatin are highly emetogenic. Almost all chemotherapy regimens include prophylactic antiemetics and patients are given oral antiemetics to take home and this usually includes 72 hours of oral dexamethasone 4 mg BD. Early management is of importance as protracted nausea and vomiting could lead to renal failure. This includes the following:

- Domperidone 10 mg TDS PO or metoclopramide 10 mg TDS IV if the patient is unable to swallow
- Ondansetron 4–8 mg BD or granisetron 3 mg IV for acute or delayed emesis
- If symptoms persist, consider third-line agents such as haloperidol 1.5 mg PO/SC every night as well as metoclopramide 30–60 mg/24 hour given via a syringe driver
- IV fluids will be required if significant reduction in oral intake is reported. After discussing with the oncologist, stop anticancer therapy in moderate to severe cases of emesis
- Be mindful of other causes of emesis – e.g. electrolyte disturbance, bowel obstruction, causes related to the underlying disease.

Neutropenic sepsis

Neutropenia is defined as follows:

- Mild neutropenia: absolute neutrophil count 1000–1500 μL

- Moderate neutropenia: absolute neutrophil count 500–1000 μL
- Severe neutropenia: absolute neutrophil count < 500 μL

The absolute neutrophil count is 6000 μL if the whole cell count is 10,000 /μL and 60% are neutrophils.

All patients who have received any chemotherapeutic agent within 6 weeks are at risk of neutropenic sepsis that could be fatal. Patients may be critically ill with minimal signs and in cases of profound neutropenia may not mount a pyrexia:

- Obtaining a focused history and perform an examination to try and identify a source. Often the source of infection is unidentifiable
- Appropriate investigations include urgent FBC, U&E, LFT, clotting screen, CRP, lactate, serum glucose, blood cultures – peripheral and from central venous access devices. Other cultures as dictated by history and examination findings
- Commence IV antibiotics according to local protocol – this should be administered within 1 hour of patient arrival. Do not wait for confirmatory FBC result. A typical regime would be tazocin 4.5 g QDS plus gentamicin
- IV fluids to maintain urine output of 30 mL/min, oxygen to maintain 94% saturation
- Early appropriate referral to critical care departments in patients should be made; especially in those who are receiving neoadjuvant chemotherapy with an aim to proceed to curative surgery or chemoradiotherapy or those undergoing curative or adjuvant treatment

Chemotherapy in practice

Induction chemotherapy

Chemotherapy administered prior to definitive treatment of locally advanced disease downstages the disease, thereby improving the chance of cure while eliminating micrometastases. As surgical and radiation techniques improve, rates of loco-regional control have also improved. There is now an increased focus on reduction of the rates of metastatic disease by way of induction chemotherapy.

Evidence exists to support the role of cisplatin and 5FU in this setting (Monnerat et al. 2002). More recently, the addition of docetaxel has shown further improvements in local control and increase in survival (Posner et al. 2007, Vermorken et al. 2007). A typical regime used in clinical practice is TPF: docetaxel 75 mg/m^2 day 1, cisplatin 75 mg/m^2 day 1 and 5FU 1000 mg/m^2 day 1–4, every 3 weeks. Response is assessed after two cycles with a maximum of three cycles administered. A note is required about nasopharyngeal carcinomas: this disease subsite was not studied in the latter two trials and therefore cisplatin and 5FU remain the regime of choice here.

Increased rates of organ preservation are observed when induction TPF is used in locally advanced laryngeal cancers.

The question of induction chemotherapy versus primary concurrent chemoradiotherapy is currently under investigation.

Concurrent chemotherapy with radiotherapy

In unresectable locally advanced malignancies, or in cases were organ preservation is sought, concurrent chemoradiotherapy is the treatment of choice. Soo et al. (2005) compared combination chemoradiotherapy with surgery and adjuvant radiotherapy in patients with stage III/IV non-metastatic head and neck cancer (non-nasopharyngeal, non-salivary). Results revealed no difference in disease free or overall survival at 6 years median follow-up. The overall organ preservation rate was 45% and higher rates were observed in laryngeal and hypopharyngeal lesions. The study has been criticized as it was not statistically powered to detect small differences in disease free or overall survival rates between the two arms.

There is robust evidence supporting the role of concurrent cisplatin with primary radiotherapy. Pignon's meta-analysis (2000) reported an additional 8% survival benefit. Cisplatin is a potent radiosensitizer – in this context, it acts by inhibiting three of the five Rs of radiobiology: repair of sublethal DNA radiation damage, repopulation of malignant cells, reoxygenation by preferentially killing hypoxic cells as well as killing micrometastases.

Patient selection is important as there is a significant increase in treatment-related toxicities. A good performance status (0–1) is required as well as ensuring a thorough past medical history has been obtained.

The dosing schedule commonly used is cisplatin 100 mg/m^2 on week 1, 4, and 7. Increasingly, weekly cisplatin (40 mg/m^2) for 6 weeks is being used as it is better tolerated.

Adjuvant chemoradiotherapy

Patients with positive surgical resection margins and evidence of extra-capsular spread in pathologically involved nodes are at particular risk of loco-regional disease recurrence.

Two recent trials have demonstrated the benefit of chemotherapy in the postoperative setting. The RTOG study (Copper et al. 2004) and EORTC study (Bernier et al. 2004) both demonstrated a reduction in rates of loco-regional disease recurrence. The latter study also suggested an improvement in overall survival.

The chemotherapeutic agent of choice is cisplatin, typically at 100 mg/m^2, 3 weekly. Its mode of action is as described for primary concurrent chemoradiotherapy.

Palliative chemotherapy

The main role of chemotherapy in this setting is to reduce the bulk of disease and consequently improve symptoms. Objective response rates have been recorded at approximately 30% of cases. A combination of cisplatin and 5FU is considered to be first-line treatment. Carboplatin can be substituted for cisplatin if GFR < 40 mL/min. Increasingly, the addition of cetuximab to the chemotherapy is being used as a minor improvement in overall survival has been reported. This is discussed below.

Sadly, the response rate of second-line therapies is disappointing (< 10%). Agents under evaluation include taxanes, gemcitabine, capecitabine, and targeted therapies.

Although response to palliative chemotherapy is moderate and short lived, any response may produce a significant improvement in the patient's quality of life.

EGFR inhibition

EGFR is a tyrosine kinase transmembrane protein involved in cell signaling and growth. The epidermal growth factor (EGF) binds to EGFR, initiating signaling cascade. Abnormally activated EGFR has been shown to be associated with carcinogenesis. A significant number of head and neck malignancies overexpress EGFR and this confers a poorer prognosis. Inhibition of apparently activated EGFR signaling cascade has been exploited in the treatment of malignancies.

Cetuximab is a recombinant chimeric (mouse-human) monoclonal antibody that binds with high affinity to human EGFR and inhibits growth, promotes apoptosis and decreases vascular endothelial growth receptor production.

Bonner et al. (2006) showed a statistically significant improvement in overall survival when cetuximab was combined with radiotherapy versus radiotherapy alone (54 months vs. 28 months $p = 0.02$). Criticisms have been made, however, as the study was not compared to concurrent chemoradiotherapy. NICE recommends the use of concurrent cetuximab-radiotherapy in patients who have contra-indications to cisplatin (e.g. poor renal function and ototoxicity). It is given intravenously as a loading dose 1-week preradiotherapy with weekly infusions during the radiotherapy course.

It also has a role in the palliative setting – the extreme study showed that its addition to cisplatin and 5FU improved overall survival compared to chemotherapy alone. Further agents are also under evaluation looking at EGFR1 and EGFR2 inhibition.

Common and important toxicities include infusion-related reactions, acneiform rash, diarrhea, stomatitis, nausea and vomiting, headaches, interstitial pneumonitis, and electrolyte disturbance including hypomagnesemia and hypokalemia:

- Research is currently underway into the role of bevacizumab in nasopharyngeal carcinomas. The RTOG 0615 study is exploring whether the addition of this targeted agent to concurrent chemoradiotherapy can reduce the risk of distant metastasis. Bevacizumab is a humanized monoclonal antibody that selectively binds to human VEGF, reducing tumor vascularization, thereby inhibiting tumor growth. There are serious comorbidities associated with bevacizumab that include arterial thromboembolic events, gastrointestinal perforation, fistula and intra-abdominal abscesses, hemorrhages, hypertension proteinuria, and necrotizing fasciitis.

Summary

Non-surgical management of head and neck cancers is increasingly adopted. Where chemotherapy and radiotherapy were once the preserve of unresectable and palliative cases only, non-surgical oncological management has become an important component for the treatment of this group of patients.

Systemic therapy is an important part of a multimodality approach in the treatment of locally advanced malignancies. Palliative chemotherapy has an important role in improving symptoms and subsequently quality of life in what can be debilitating recurrent or metastatic disease.

In the neoadjuvant setting, chemotherapy may reduce the likelihood of distant metastases while improving the locoregional control provided by definitive surgery or radiotherapy. Primary concurrent chemotherapy improves overall survival when compared to radiotherapy alone in locally advanced disease. In patients for whom cisplatin is contraindicated, cetuximab is licensed by NICE for use in combination with radiotherapy. For patients with positive resection margins or evidence of extracapsular spread in malignant lymphadenopathy, addition of chemotherapy to adjuvant radiotherapy reduces the rate of loco-regional disease recurrence.

Research into using cetuximab with both primary concurrent chemoradiotherapy and post op chemoradiotherapy is underway. The RTOG 0522 trial looked at the addition of cetuximab to concurrent chemotherapy plus accelerated radiotherapy in stages III–IV head and neck squamous carcinomas – there was no improvement of either progression-free or overall survival. Future studies will continue to evaluate the role of biological agents with more advanced radiation techniques.

References

Bernier J, Domenge C, Ozsahin M, et al. Post-operative irradiation with or without concomitant chemotherapy for locally advanced head and neck cancer patients. N Engl J Med 2004; 350:1945–52.

Bonner J, Harari P, Giralt J, et al. Radiotherapy plus cetuximab for squamous cell carcinoma of the head and neck. N Engl J Med 2006; 354:567–78.

Cooper J, Pajak T, Forastiere A, et al. Postoperative concurrent radiotherapy and chemotherapy for high-risk squamous cell carcinoma of the head and neck. N Engl J Med 2004; 350:1937–44.

Monnerat C, Faivre S, Teman S, et al. End points for new agents in induction chemotherapy for locally advanced cancers. Ann Oncol 2002; 13:995–1006.

Pignon JP, Bourhis J, Domenge C, et al. Chemotherapy added to locoregional treatment for head and neck squamous cell carcinoma: three meta-analyses of updated individual data. MACH-NC Collaborative Group. Meta-analysis of chemotherapy on Head and Neck cancer. Lancet 2000; 355:949–55.

Posner M, Hershock D, Blajman C, et al. Cisplatin and fluorouracil alone or with docetaxel in head and neck cancer. N Engl J Med 2007; 357:1705–15.

Soo KC, Tan EH, Wee J, et al. Surgery and adjuvant radiotherapy vs. concurrent chemoradiotherapy in stage III/IV non-metastatic squamous cell head and neck cancer: a randomised comparison. Br J Cancer 2005; 93:279–86.

Vermorken J, Remenar E, van Herpen C, et al. Cisplatin fluorouracil and docetaxel in unresectable head and neck cancer. N Engl J Med 2007; 357:1695–704.

Mymoona Alzouebi and Martin H. Robinson

Radiotherapy remains the most effective non-surgical modality in the treatment of cancer. In recent years, radiotherapy has witnessed rapid technological advances in the delivery of sophisticated treatments to a range of cancers in a multitude of disease sites. However, the basic principles of radiotherapy remain unchanged. The objective of radiotherapy is to kill cancer cells while limiting damage to surrounding normal tissue.

The therapeutic effect of radiotherapy is achieved through tumor cell apoptosis with the key molecular target being cellular DNA. Damage occurs directly by inducing breaks in the DNA helical structure and indirectly by the production of unstable, highly reactive free radicals that also damage the DNA. In addition, radiation can also directly ionize DNA, leading to direct damage of the DNA's bases or sugar phosphate backbone.

Radiation-induced damage can either be lethal (irreversible causing cell death) or sublethal where the damage may be repaired. The probability of lethal cell injury depends on the type and amount of radiation administered. This together with the biological factors that influence normal tissue and tumor responses to radiotherapy can be summarized in the five 'Rs' of radiobiology: Radiosensitivity, Reoxygenation, Redistribution, Repopulation, and Repair.

The radiosensitivity of cells varies throughout the cell cycle. Cells are most vulnerable in the G2/M phase of the cycle presumably due to having little time to repair radiation induced damage before division and least vulnerable in the S phase. Therefore, within a given tumor, individual cells are in different phases of the cell cycle and hence radiosensitivity can vary. Redistribution occurs when cells in the more radiosensitive phases of the cell cycle (M/G2) die off and the surviving cells redistribute into the more sensitive phases of the cycle. Subsequent fractions of radiation may then be more efficient at killing these cells.

In addition, it is widely accepted that hypoxia also results in radioresistance and poor radiotherapy outcomes. This is because tumors often have a chaotic vasculature which, when coupled with limited diffusion of oxygen in an often highly proliferative tumor, results in areas of chronic hypoxia and nutrient deprivation. Consequently, due to the lack of molecular oxygen reacting with the induced DNA radicals to produce irreparable damage anoxic or hypoxic cells are considerably more resistant to the lethal effects of radiation than oxic cells. Therefore, it is important for patients undergoing radical radiotherapy treatments to have reasonable hemoglobin concentrations to facilitate oxygenation of tumors.

The majority of cell damage induced by radiation is sublethal and can be repaired, leading to increased cell survival. Most of the repair in normal tissues occurs within 6 hours of radiation exposure, therefore if a second dose of radiation is given during this period, there is increased risk of normal tissue damage. Provided adequate time for repair between doses is given a greater overall dose of radiation can be delivered with sparing of normal tissues. Therefore, fractionation of treatment leads to much less late radiation-induced tissue damage.

The final radiobiological principle, repopulation, may occur during prolonged courses of radiotherapy or where treatment is protracted as a consequence of toxicity. It is most likely to occur in well to moderately differentiated tumors with large growth fractions and short cell cycle times and is particularly relevant in head and neck cancers.

Radiotherapy in practice

The dose of radiation is prescribed as units of gray (Gy) – a measure of the total absorbed radiation energy (1 Gy = 1 joule per kilogram (J/Kg)) – and is delivered in a number of individual fractions.

Radiation can be produced both naturally from radioactive isotopes or artificially and is delivered in three main ways:

1. **External beam radiotherapy:** This involves treating patients with beams of radiation produced from a source external to the patient. The Linear accelerator machine can produce very high-energy megavoltage X-rays (photons) and electrons (**Figure 5.1**). Electrons are very useful for treating superficial tumors and can spare underlying tissues such as the spinal cord. Photons, on the other hand, provide better tissue penetration. In addition, the design of the machine allows treatment of the patient at any angle.

2. **Brachytherapy:** This is the placement of radioactive sources within tumors (interstitial) or body cavities (intracavitary). It allows high doses of radiation to be delivered directly to the tumor and sparing nearby structures due to the rapid fall off in the dose with increasing distance from the source. Those used include iridium 192, iodine 125, and cesium 137.

3. **Systemic isotope therapy:** This involves the oral or intravenous delivery of radionuclides.

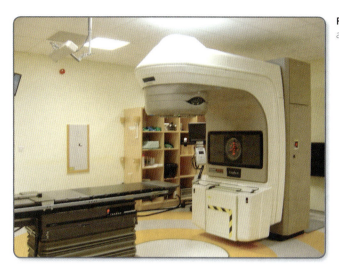

Figure 5.1 Standard linear accelerator.

Radiotherapy treatment planning

The integral steps in planning radiotherapy to the head and neck area involve a series of steps.

Preplanning

Dentition

All patients undergoing radical/curative treatments should have a full dental assessment prior to radiotherapy. Often radiotherapy treatment fields will involve part or all of the mandible and salivary glands that can lead to xerostomia and tooth decay. Any problem teeth should be removed prior to radiotherapy.

Nutrition

Specialist dietician assessment is essential for this group of patients who are often malnourished prior to treatment. Many have a background of excessive alcohol intake and may suffer impaired swallowing due to the direct effect of the tumor. Patients undergoing radical radiotherapy to the upper aerodigestive tract (UADT) over several weeks develop severe mucositis and dysphagia that can significantly reduce their oral intake and weight. A radiologically inserted gastrostomy or a percutaneous gastrostomy should be considered in all patients whose UADT mucosa will be included in the radiation field, indeed they merit consideration in any patient undergoing chemoradiation treatment that incorporates a wide field.

Audiometry

This should be considered in patients undergoing concurrent chemoradiation with the use of cisplatin, known to be ototoxic.

Smoking cessation

Smoking is associated with 85–90% of head and neck malignancies. Patients should be actively encouraged to stop smoking and appropriately supported. It is accepted that continued smoking during and after treatment increases toxicity from radiotherapy and also increases the subsequent risk of recurrence and second primary cancers.

Immobilization

It is essential that radiation treatment is reproducible on a daily basis in order to minimize the risk of geographical misses, optimize tumor control, and reduce excess damage to normal tissues. This is best achieved by immobilization of the area treated and is of significant importance in head and neck cancers because of the close proximity of critical structures such as spinal cord. Typically patients will have a custom made plastic/thermoplastic head shell prior to treatment (**Figure 5.2**). A mouth bite may be necessary when treating cancers of the tongue or floor of mouth allowing displacement of the upper jaw out of the treatment field.

Localization

It is the role of the treating oncologist in identifying the site of the tumor and the 'at risk' areas. This must take into account all the clinical (examination/endoscopy), radiological (MRI/PET) and pathological data. Patients will undergo a planning CT scan immobilized in the treatment position to increase reproducibility. The gross tumor volume (GTV) and the predicted subclinical spread of disease (Clinical Target Volume – CTV) is delineated on the CT scan using a treatment planning system. In order to make sure that the entire CTV receives the prescribed dose, a further margin is required to account for day-to-day variations due to patient and organ movement: this larger volume is known as the planning target volume (PTV). Organs at risk such as spinal cord, brainstem and parotid glands should also be defined in order to assess the doses received by these structures.

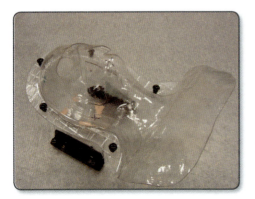
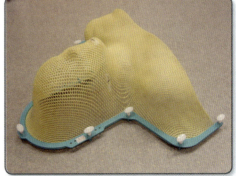

Figure 5.2 Examples of immobilization head shells.

Planning

Once the treatment volume (GTV, CTV, and PTV) and organs at risk are delineated, the radiotherapy planners or physicists then use a 3D planning system to define the correct radiotherapy technique to deliver the treatment (**Figure 5.3**). This takes into account beam arrangement, beam energy, size, shape, and weighting in addition to the use of wedges to compensate for sloping external surfaces or to even out dose. A 'plan' is then produced that displays the dose distribution across the treatment volume and normal structures. A DVH (dose volume histogram) showing the proportion of the volume of any structure that receives a specified dose of radiation is also produced by the planning system (**Figure 5.4**). The oncologist reviews the plan and the DVH to ensure that the tumor is being treated adequately while sparing normal tissues as much as possible.

Verification

To ensure the accuracy of treatment, check X-ray films are taken prior to and during radiotherapy. Most linear accelerators now have portal imaging systems that utilize computer software programs to produce images of the treated area from the therapy beams view to help assess for deviations of the treatment from that which was intended.

Radiotherapy techniques

3D conformal radiotherapy

This is the standard technique explained above which incorporates the use of CT images to facilitate conformal shaping of the treatment volumes, optimization of beam direction and weighting.

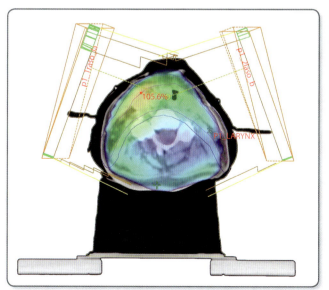

Figure 5.3 Conventional 3D conformal radiotherapy plan for laryngeal cancer treating bilateral necks as well.

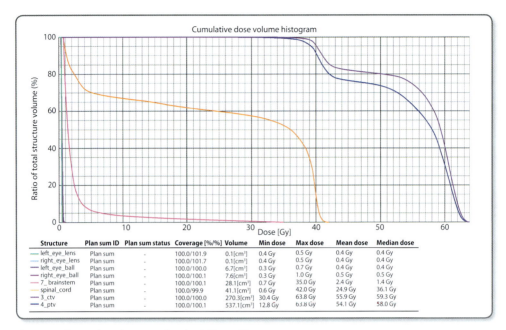

Structure	Plan sum ID	Plan sum status	Coverage [%/%]	Volume	Min dose	Max dose	Mean dose	Median dose
left_eye_lens	Plan sum	-	100.0/101.9	0.1[cm³]	0.4 Gy	0.5 Gy	0.4 Gy	0.4 Gy
right_eye_lens	Plan sum	-	100.0/101.7	0.1[cm³]	0.4 Gy	0.5 Gy	0.4 Gy	0.4 Gy
left_eye_ball	Plan sum	-	100.0/100.0	6.7[cm³]	0.3 Gy	0.7 Gy	0.4 Gy	0.4 Gy
right_eye_ball	Plan sum	-	100.0/100.1	7.6[cm³]	0.3 Gy	1.0 Gy	0.5 Gy	0.5 Gy
7_brainstem	Plan sum	-	100.0/100.1	28.1[cm³]	0.7 Gy	35.0 Gy	2.4 Gy	1.4 Gy
spinal_cord	Plan sum	-	100.0/99.9	41.1[cm³]	0.6 Gy	42.0 Gy	24.9 Gy	36.1 Gy
3_ctv	Plan sum	-	100.0/100.0	270.3[cm³]	30.4 Gy	63.8 Gy	55.9 Gy	59.3 Gy
4_ptv	Plan sum	-	100.0/100.1	537.1[cm³]	12.8 Gy	63.8 Gy	54.1 Gy	58.0 Gy

Figure 5.4 Dose volume histogram for plan in Figure 5.3.

Intensity-modulated radiotherapy

This is a type of conformal radiotherapy that allows optimization of the dose delivered to the target volume and minimizes the dose delivered to critical structures (**Figure 5.5**). The intensity of the beam is varied across the treatment field, allowing a single beam to function as a number of smaller beams, facilitating coverage of complex and especially concave target volumes thus producing an overall highly conformal plan. It also allows spontaneous boost doses to be given to areas of high risk/residual disease and avoids dose-limiting normal tissues. It should be the standard in nasopharyngeal and parotid cancer. The planning of intensity modulated radiotherapy is, however, labor intensive.

Image-guided radiotherapy

This technique seeks to further increase the accuracy and reproducibility of the treatment plan by daily imaging of, in the case of head and neck cancers, bone and soft tissues to correct and check 'on-line' the treatment before delivery. This increased imaging therefore facilitates the reduction in margins from CTV to PTV, hence reducing overall treatment volume.

Indications for radiotherapy in head and neck cancer

Radiotherapy can be used as a single modality treatment or as a multimodality treatment with surgery. It can be used in four main ways:
1. Radical curative radiotherapy (alone or in combination with chemotherapy)

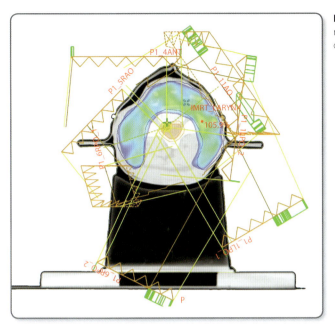

Figure 5.5 Intensity modulated radiotherapy plan for laryngeal cancer.

2. Postoperative adjuvant radiotherapy (alone or in combination with chemotherapy)
3. Brachytherapy
4. Palliative radiotherapy

Radical curative radiotherapy (alone or in combination with chemotherapy)

The choice of the primary treatment modality depends on tumor site and accessibility, stage and operability, pathological subtype, functional outcome and the patients' performance status and wishes. Assessment at the multidisciplinary team meeting is essential. More than 60% of squamous head and neck cancer present with advanced locoregional disease and while surgery should always be considered, often it is technically not possible or would be associated with unacceptable morbidity, e.g. base of tongue cancer requiring glossectomy and consequent loss of swallow and voice. Alternatively, significant comorbidity and high operative risk may preclude patients from a surgical approach.

The use of chemotherapy concurrently with radiotherapy is associated with a modest improvement in survival over radiotherapy alone (4–8% increase in 5-year survival) (Bernier et al. 2004, Bonner et al. 2006). The most commonly used drug is single-agent cisplatin, although cetuximab can be considered in patients intolerant of cisplatin (Calais et al. 1999). Combined modality therapy is associated with increased toxicity, in particular mucositis, and therefore should only be considered in patients with good performance status and normal renal function.

Primary radiotherapy or chemoradiotherapy can be considered in the following circumstances:

- Early laryngeal cancer (T1 and T2) similar control rates are seen with endoscopic laryngeal surgery and radiotherapy
- T3 laryngeal cancer is a heterogeneous group and can be treated with primary chemoradiotherapy and salvage surgery or laryngectomy and post op radiotherapy
- Oropharyngeal cancers are largely treated with chemoradiotherapy unless early stage and well lateralized when surgery may be considered
- Hypopharyngeal cancers are often treated with a combination of surgery and post op radiotherapy or primary chemoradiotherapy if organ preservation is a possibility
- Nasopharyngeal cancers due to their surgical inaccessibility are best treated with chemoradiotherapy
- Where the patients choice or physical state precludes surgery

Total dose is 66–70 Gy in 1.8–2 Gy per fraction treating Monday to Friday over 6.5/7 weeks.

Postoperative radiotherapy (alone or in combination with chemotherapy)

The goal of postoperative radiotherapy is to improve loco-regional control. It is also accepted that cancer specific and overall survival can be improved as a consequence (Garden et al. 2004, Lavaf et al. 2008). The indications for postoperative radiotherapy can be divided into tumor-related factors or nodal factors, with asterisk (*) identifying absolute indications. Treatment should ideally commence as soon as possible after surgery provided the wound has healed and the patients' fitness allows, typically within 6 weeks.

Tumor factors

- Positive (involved) resection margins*
- Close resection margin (< 5 mm)
- T3–T4 primary tumor
- Perineural or perivascular invasion
- Multicentric primary
- High grade/poorly differentiated

Nodal factors

- Extracapsular spread*
- ≥ 2 nodes involved
- > 1 nodal level
- Involved node > 3 cm in diameter, i.e. ≥ N2 disease

The addition of chemotherapy, namely, cisplatin should be considered in patients with high-risk pathological features following surgical resection of oral cavity, oropharyngeal, laryngeal or hypopharyngeal cancers.

Total dose is 50–60 Gy in 2 Gy per fraction treating Monday to Friday over 5/6 weeks. An additional boost of 6 Gy can be given to areas with suspected residual microscopic disease.

Brachytherapy

Cross-network service provision for highly specialized brachytherapy treatment should be available. In general, brachytherapy can be considered for:

- Small lesions, ideally < 3 cm
- Accessible tumors, e.g. oral cavity and oropharyngeal
- Tumors not attached or in close proximity to bone
- Tumors with no nodal involvement

The GEC-ESTRO recommendations produced in 2009 provide a comprehensive outline of patients suitable for brachytherapy (Mazeron et al. 2009).

Palliative radiotherapy

Applying the same principles, radiotherapy can be used to provide symptom control in patients unfit for radical treatments. Common indications include pain, dysphagia, and bleeding (Stevens et al. 2011). However, the pros of such treatment must outweigh the potential risks/side effects.

Toxicity of radiotherapy

Side effects of radiotherapy to the head and neck area usually begin after about 2 weeks of treatment. Initially, patients present with mild soreness in the mouth and throat, particularly worse on swallowing. This progresses as treatment continues until 2 weeks or so after radiotherapy ends. Radiotherapy side effects are considerably worse when concurrent chemotherapy is used.

Acute

- Mucositis
- Dysphagia: secondary to mucositis, loss of taste and appetite and due to thickened secretions
- Skin reaction: erythema, dry desquamation, moist desquamation, ulceration
- Fatigue

Late

- Skin pigmentation/atrophy
- Alopecia in the areas treated
- Xerostomia: arises primarily due to radiotherapy to the parotid gland and to a lesser degree the submandibular and sublingual glands
- Osteoradionecrosis: breakdown of bone within the treatment volume, most commonly seen in the mandible

Care of the head and neck patient

Patients should have regular clinical reviews, ideally weekly, during radiotherapy with the appropriate input given.

Mouth care: regular mouth washes and saline rinses, dental hygiene with regular teeth brushing.

Skin care: regular emollient cream application. If skin becomes broken, a barrier product should be used.

Dietetic care: regular review by dietician with implementation of nutritional supplements and gastrostomy feeds.

Pain: analgesics used should comprise soluble paracetamol, co-codamol or alcohol free liquid morphine. Occasionally, patients may need to be admitted to optimize pain control.

Summary

Radiotherapy for head and neck cancers can be a sole treatment or can be a component of a multimodality therapy with surgery and chemotherapy. The choice of treatment modality depends on tumor site, stage, operability, patient's performance status and wishes, functional outcome and cosmesis. Assessment in a multidisciplinary clinic is essential.

Further reading

Bomford CK, Kunkler IH. Walter and Miller's Textbook of Radiotherapy: Radiation Physics, Therapy, and Oncology . London: Churchill Livingstone, 2003.

Lindberg R. Distribution of cervical lymph node metastases from squamous cell carcinoma of the upper respiratory and digestive tracts. Cancer 1972; 29:1446–9.

Chao KS, Wippold FJ, Ozyigit G, et al. Determination and delineation of nodal target volumes for head-and-neck cancer based on patterns of failure in patients receiving definitive and postoperative IMRT. Int J Radiat Oncol Biol Phys 2002; 53:1174–84.

Gregoire V, Ang K, Budach W, et al. Delineation of the neck node levels for head and neck tumors: a 2013 update. Philadelphia, PA: Radiation Therapy Oncology Group, 2013 (online)

References

Bernier J, Domenge C, Ozsahin M, et al. Postoperative irradiation with or without concomitant chemotherapy for locally advanced head and neck cancer. N Engl J Med 2004; 350:1945–52.

Bonner JA, Harari PM, Giralt J, et al. Radiotherapy plus cetuximab for squamous-cell carcinoma of the head and neck N Engl J Med 2006; 354:567–78.

Calais G, Alfonsi M, Bardet E, et al. Randomized trial of radiation therapy versus concomitant chemotherapy and radiation therapy for advanced-stage oropharynx carcinoma. J Natl Cancer Inst 1999; 91:2081–6.

Garden AS, Harris J, Vokes EE, et al. Preliminary results of Radiation Therapy Oncology Group 97-03: a randomized phase ii trial of concurrent radiation and chemotherapy for advanced squamous cell carcinomas of the head and neck. J Clin Oncol 2004; 22:2856–64.

Lavaf A, Genden EM, Cesaretti JA, et al. Adjuvant radiotherapy improves overall survival for patients with lymph node-positive head and neck squamous cell carcinoma. Cancer 2008; 112:535–43.

Mazeron JJ, Ardiet JM, Haie-Méder C, et al. GEC-ESTRO recommendations for brachytherapy for head and neck squamous cell carcinomas. Radiother Oncol 2009; 91:150–56.

Stevens CM, Huang SH, Fung S, et al. Retrospective study of palliative radiotherapy in newly diagnosed head and neck carcinoma. Int J Radiat Oncol Biol Phys 2011; 81:958–63.

Radical neck dissection

Nicholas Stafford

The radical neck dissection (RND), and subsequent modifications of it, has been a cornerstone of head and neck oncology since Crile pioneered the operation in 1906.

In the vast majority of cases, the neck is the first site a primary head and neck squamous carcinoma metastasizes to. Certainly, in cases of squamous cancer appropriate management of the neck is crucial for optimum survival. It is known that:

- Neck metastasis reduces the patient's prognosis for a particular stage primary head and neck squamous cell carcinoma (HNSCC) by approximately 50%
- Multiple level nodal metastases and extracapsular lymph node spread (both requiring histopathological assessment) also have a profound effect on prognosis

Therefore, an active approach to the management of the neck can have a significant effect on patient survival.

Neck levels

Six levels have been described. They are demonstrated in **Figure 6.1.**

Level 1: Submental and submandibular nodes
Level 2: Upper deep cervical chain nodes (around internal jugular vein down to level of hyoid bone)
Level 3: Mid deep cervical chain nodes (around internal jugular vein from hyoid bone to cricoid cartilage level)
Level 4: Lower deep cervical chain nodes (below level of cricoid cartilage)
Level 5: Posterior triangle nodes (primarily around accessory nerve and transverse cervical artery)
Level 6: Lymph nodes lying anterior to the midline visceral structures

Over the second half of the last century variations of the classical radical neck dissection were developed, with the intention of preserving

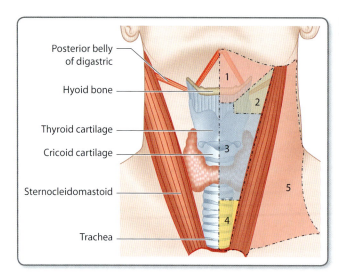

Figure 6.1 The five clinical levels of the cervical nodes.

Posterior belly of digastric

Hyoid bone

Thyroid cartilage

Cricoid cartilage

Sternocleidomastoid

Trachea

structure and function and thereby reducing morbidity where possible. In 1991, a classification of such procedures was formulated:

1. Radical neck dissection: clearance of levels 1–5 with sacrifice of the sternomastoid muscle, internal jugular vein and accessory nerve
2. Modified radical neck dissection: clearance of levels 1–5 but with preservation of one or more of the three structures sacrificed in a radical dissection
3. Selective neck dissection: clearance of less than all five lymph node groups mentioned above. Traditionally, four types are described:
   a. Supraomohyoid: levels 1–3 are cleared
   b. Posteriolateral: levels 2–5 are cleared
   c. Lateral: levels 2–4 are cleared
   d. Anterior: level 6 cleared
4. Extended radical neck dissection: removal of lymph node levels 1–5, the sternomastoid muscle, accessory nerve and internal jugular vein and one of more other structures or lymph node groups.

Preoperative considerations

Where possible, clinical assessment of the neck should be augmented by appropriate imaging. Generally speaking, MRI is preferable to CT scanning but the later can be indicated in specific situations. Ultrasound, with fine needle guided aspiration, is particularly useful in delineating metastases in small, sometimes impalpable, nodes.

Angiography is rarely necessary but may be indicated if carotid resection and replacement is feasible. Such a situation is very unusual: involvement of the artery is usually accompanied by other evidence of extensive disease.

In general, tumor invasion of the common or internal carotid artery, the brachial plexus, or the prevertebral musculature indicates such aggressive disease as to contra-indicate surgery. Likewise, extension of the lymph node mass below the level of the clavicle usually renders the neck inoperable.

Having decided to proceed with a neck dissection the next consideration is which type to undertake. Indications for the various types are shown in **Table 6.1**.

Preservation of the sternomastoid muscle is really just for cosmetic purposes. However, if the neck disease is not too extensive, an attempt should be made to preserve the accessory nerve if it is distant from macroscopic disease. Postoperative morbidity after nerve sacrifice can be significant, particularly in the manual worker whose dominant side nerve has been removed.

Preserve the internal jugular vein. This is particularly important where there is a significant chance of subsequent contralateral neck disease. The morbidity resulting from the loss of both veins is considerable

Consent for surgery

It is essential that the patient is made aware of the possible complications and the likely long-term morbidities associated with the operation (e.g. bleeding, frozen shoulder, and paraesthesia).

Table 6.1 Indications for the various types of neck dissection					
Radical neck dissection	**Modified radical neck dissection**	**Supraomohyoid neck dissection**	**Lateral neck dissection**	**Posterolateral neck dissection**	**Extended neck dissection**
A large solitary cervical node (6 cm diameter +) or multiple lymph node metastases, where the IJV, XI nerve and sternomastoid muscle cannot be safely preserved	Clinically evident nodal disease where the internal jugular vein and/or accessory nerve can be safely preserved: levels 1-5 are resected	Clinical node negative cases of oral squamous cell carcinoma	Clinically node negative squamous cell carcinoma of the larynx, oropharynx, or hypopharynx	Clinically node positive neck with laryngeal or hypopharyngeal primary	Removal of structures such as prevertebral musculature, XII nerve, carotid artery (with reconstruction where indicated)
		Single small mobile level 1 or 2 node from oral cavity, lip or facial skin		Cutaneous scalp malignancies	Resection of paratracheal nodes in continuity with neck dissection (e.g. postcricoid, thyroid cancers)
					Resection of retropharyngeal nodes where accessible (e.g. usually from oropharyngeal or hypopharyngeal primary)

Antibiotics

Prophylactic antibiotics are not necessary if the mucosa of the upper aerodigestive tract is not breached.

Incisions

Avoid a three part junction if possible, particularly in the postradiation neck. Variations on the utility, apron, incision are usually adequate (**Figure 6.2**). These incisions can be modified depending on whether any other procedure is being undertaken. For instance, the lateral limb of the Gluck incision employed for a laryngectomy can be taken more laterally and extended up to the mastoid process for an ipsilateral neck dissection.

If for reasons of previous surgery or poor viability of the neck skin a long apron incision is inadvisable, then the double horizontal McFee–Grillo incision is a safe standby.

Operative technique

Exposure

- The skin flaps are raised in the subplatysmal plane, extending to the anterior edge of trapezius, the horizontal ramus of the mandible, the anterior midline/strap muscles and the clavicle
- The external jugular vein is divided and tied superiorly and inferiorly

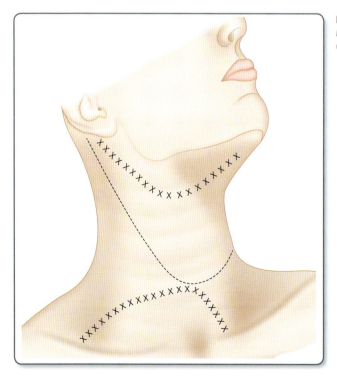

Figure 6.2 Double horizontal, McFee–Grillo (×××××) and utility (- - - - -) incisions.

- The lower end of the sternomastoid muscle is divided about 1 cm above its insertion into the clavicle and manubrium. This can be safely undertaken using cutting diathermy (**Figure 6.3**)

The inferior dissection

- The lower end of the internal jugular vein is then located by careful dissection and opening of the carotid sheath. The vein is dissected out, with adequate access to its medial and lateral walls, for about 2–3 cm. This allows it to be safely tied and divided, having first ensured that the vagus nerve has not been picked up with the vein. Suture ligation of the vein can also be employed but be careful not to tear the vein with the needle. Unless necessitated by the site of the lymph node mass, do not divide the vein too low, i.e. behind the clavicle. Losing control of the lower end of the vein can result in a catastrophic air embolus
- Check that the lymphatic duct has not been damaged. Look for a chyle leak (this is more likely to be apparent during/after a left-sided procedure)
- Having secured the lower end of the vein start to develop the plane of dissection between it and the vagus nerve and carotid artery. Work up the anterior aspect of the vein, maintaining a 'broad front' along the plane of the dissection
- Divide the soft tissues just above the clavicle, parallel to its upper border, moving laterally from the tied end of the internal jugular vein
- Divide the clavicular insertion of the omohyoid muscle

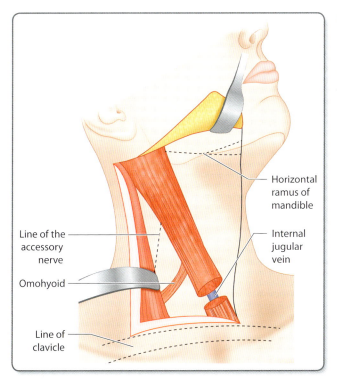

Figure 6.3 A utility incision has been employed and the skin flaps raised. The lower end of the sternomastoid muscle has been divided to expose the internal jugular vein.

Horizontal ramus of mandible

Line of the accessory nerve

Internal jugular vein

Omohyoid

Line of clavicle

- Use blunt dissection, e.g. a swab wrapped round a finger, to push the supraclavicular soft tissues superiorly. Identify and divide the suprascapular vessels. Having created this important plane of dissection on the prevertebral fascia, identify the brachial plexus and phrenic nerve (the latter running over the surface of scalenus anterior)
- Continue the dissection laterally to the anterior border of trapezius. Then, on a broad front, elevate the whole specimen superiorly, working up trapezius and the carotid tree and vagus nerve in parallel
- About a third of the way up the anterior border of trapezius, the accessory nerve will be encountered. This is sectioned at this point in a radial neck dissection
- At the level of the hyoid bone follow the anterior belly of digastric up to the mentum. (It is only necessary to clear the submental triangle in cases of lip, anterior floor of mouth and nasal vestibule cancer)

The superior dissection

- Clear the submandibular triangle anteroposteriorly, taking care to preserve the marginal mandibular, hypoglossal, and lingual nerves. The facial vessels should be divided just inferior to the ramus of the mandible (**Figure 6.3**). The facial artery is also divided posteriorly where it loops over the superior border of posterior belly of digastric. Ligation of the facial vein and superior reflection of it and the investing facia at the level of the mandible facilitates avoidance of damage to the marginal mandibular nerve (**Figure 6.4**)
- Continue the superior dissection posteriorly, taking (if necessary) the tail of the parotid gland. Use the posterior belly of digastric as a landmark for the desired depth of the dissection
- Continue to raise the dissection off the prevertebral muscles, dividing the cervical plexus near to its root, but being careful to preserve the phrenic nerve
- Follow the hypoglossal nerve posteriorly, clearing the specimen and internal jugular vein off the carotid tree, vagus and hypoglossal nerves
- Divide the upper end of the sternomastoid muscle, again using cutting diathermy, just below its insertion into the mastoid process
- Retract the specimen superoposteriorly and then with a Lagenbeck retract the posterior belly of digastric superiorly to identify and adequately expose the top end of the internal jugular vein
- Divide and tie off the upper end of the internal jugular vein taking care to avoid damaging the vagus and hypoglossal nerves. The accessory nerve is divided as it leaves the internal jugular nerve to run posteroinferiorly into the sternocleidomastoid
- Continue to clear the dissection from the trapezius muscle, raising the whole specimen superiorly
- Complete the top end of the dissection, having preserved the internal and external carotid arteries, the hypoglossal and vagus nerves (**Figure 6.5**)

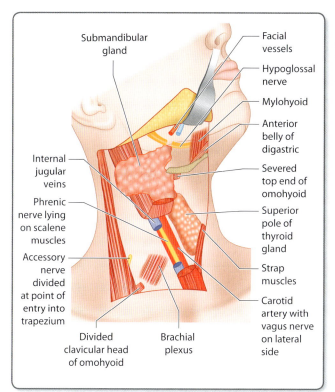

Submandibular gland

Facial vessels

Hypoglossal nerve

Mylohyoid

Anterior belly of digastric

Internal jugular veins

Severed top end of omohyoid

Phrenic nerve lying on scalene muscles

Superior pole of thyroid gland

Accessory nerve divided at point of entry into trapezium

Strap muscles

Carotid artery with vagus nerve on lateral side

Divided clavicular head of omohyoid

Brachial plexus

Figure 6.4 The lower and anterior parts of the dissection are completed. The submandibular triangle has been dissected. Dissection now needs to proceed up the carotid artery.

- Check for hematostasis. Two areas notorious for problems are the submandibular triangle (in particular, vessels related to the hypoglossal nerve) and the angle between the trapezius and lateral clavicle
- Check for chyle leak
- Close the neck after placing adequate suction drainage
  Normally skin sutures are removed at about 7 days, but they are left longer in the neck postradiotherapy.

Postoperative complications

Immediate

Damage to nerves or vascular structures will become evident in the early recovery phase. There is nothing that can be done to reverse such problems.

Significantly raised intracranial pressure can result in cerebral edema. Tying off one internal jugular vein increases intracranial pressure by a factor of three which rarely presents a management problem: the effects are very short lived. Tying both increases it by a factor of eight that can cause profound problems. This should be pre-empted by the use of prophylactic mannitol and/or diuretics.

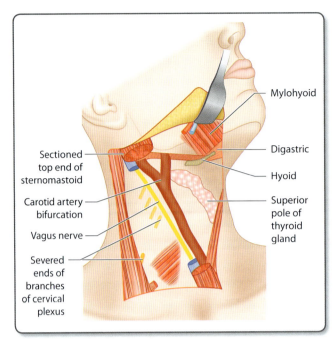

Sectioned
top end of
sternomastoid

Carotid artery
bifurcation

Vagus nerve

Severed
ends of
branches
of cervical
plexus

Mylohyoid

Digastric

Hyoid

Superior
pole of
thyroid
gland

Figure 6.5 The block dissection has been completed and the specimen removed. The anatomy of the surgical bed is demonstrated.

Early

The development of a significant hematoma occurring within the first 12 hours postoperatively will lift up the skin flaps and delay healing if it is not dealt with. If the collection is sizeable (≥ 250 mL) then the patient should be returned to theatre and the hematoma dealt with. Ensure the drains are replaced and are working correctly.

A chyle leak will usually present itself within 24–28 hours with clear fluid in the drain bottle. The fluid will become fatty/milky when feeding starts. Manage conservatively in the first instant. It will often subside. Applying pressure locally is a waste of time. Keep the local drain in situ but after 48 hours remove the suction from it. Apply a colostomy bag to the part of exit of the tube to limit skin excoriation. The patient should be kept nil by mouth and fed intravenously. If the leak exceeds 600 mL per day 7–10 days postoperatively then the wound should be re-explored and the leak stopped. The use of an operating microscope will often facilitate locating the cut end of the duct.

Wound infection is rarely serious unless it is associated with a salivary fistula. Bacteriological swabs should be taken and appropriate antibiotics should be given.

A carotid artery rupture is rare. Predisposing factors are preoperative radiotherapy to the neck and a salivary fistula. There is often a warning bleed. If this occurs or if the situation presents with a catastrophic bleed the wound needs immediate re-exploration, if possible by both a head and neck and a vascular surgeon. Immediate and adequate circulatory resuscitation is crucial if the significant chance of permanent neurological loss is to be avoided.

Late

Frozen shoulder is a serious long-term sequela, particularly for the manual worker. Physiotherapy is the only measure that helps alleviate the condition.

Specific features of modified radical and selective neck dissections

Preservation of the internal jugular vein should always be attempted where it is oncologically safe. The steps in the dissection are as outlined above, only the 'carotid tree' includes the internal jugular vein that is left in intimate contact with the common carotid artery and vagus nerve. The common facial nerve will need to be divided at its entry into the vein. Small tears in the vein can be repaired with 5.0 or 6.0 nylon.

The accessory nerve should be preserved. The nerve can be traced through and directed off the specimen either from above or below, or both. Once located at its entry into sternocleidomastoid muscle it should be carefully, tracked through the muscle. Splitting the muscle along the nerve's course will allow the latter to be kept under direct vision (as in a parotidectomy with the facial nerve). The nerve splits in the muscle: ensure that the branch to the muscle rather than the main trunk continuing to trapezius is divided. If in any doubt use a nerve stimulator.

Preservation of the sternocleidomastoid muscle is largely for cosmetic purposes and is therefore rarely undertaken. Resection of it results in insignificant functional loss.

Further reading

Robbins KT, Clayman G, Levine PA, et al. Neck dissection classification update: revisions proposed by the American Head and Neck Society and the American Academy of Otolaryngology – Head and Neck Surgery. Arch Otolaryngol Head Neck Surg 2002; 128:751–58.

Shah JP, Patel S, Singh B (eds). Jatin Shah's Head and Neck Surgery and Oncology, 4th edn. Philadelphia, PA: Mosby Elsevier; 2012.

Gavilán J, Herranz J, De Santo LW, Gavilán C (eds). Functional and Selective Neck Dissection. New York: Thieme, 2002.

Total laryngectomy

Nicholas Stafford

The first laryngectomy was performed by Bilroth in 1873. Since then it has become a mainstay of surgical treatment for cancer of the larynx.

While the last 50 years saw partial laryngectomy (vertical, horizontal, frontolateral) become popular these techniques have now been largely supplanted by per-oral endoscopic laser resection, a topic outside the scope of this book.

Total laryngectomy is now reserved for a minority of laryngeal tumors:

1. T4 lesions with involvement of the laryngeal cartilage or tumor extension beyond the confines of the laryngeal framework
2. Radioresistant tumors unsuitable for endoscopic laser resection
3. A new laryngeal tumor which lies within a previously irradiated tumor volume and which cannot be dealt with endoscopically

Preoperative considerations

While mirror or fiberoptic examination usually provides a two-dimensional assessment of the tumor, CT scanning of the larynx is the only technique that will accurately demonstrate laryngeal cartilage involvement. It will also allow assessment of cervical lymph node metastasis, although MRI or ultrasound scanning is probably superior for picking up relatively small nodal disease. A CT scan should also encompass the lungs to exclude pulmonary metastases.

All patients should undergo a formal upper aerodigestive tract endoscopy and biopsy of the primary tumor. In exceptional circumstances where the airway is acutely compromised by a large tumor, it might be appropriate to proceed immediately to total laryngectomy if a frozen section biopsy confirms carcinoma. If the tumor is obstructing the airway, but scanning suggests it is T2 or T3 in stage then laser debulking of the tumor is usually adequate in restoring a satisfactory airway prior to chemoradiotherapy.

Removal of the larynx is a psychologically devastating procedure for many patients. Preoperative counseling is therefore essential. It is vital that the patient is prepared for the inevitable tracheostomy and tube management which will be important, certainly in the short term. If possible, the patient should be introduced to an established laryngectomee prior to surgery.

Surgical voice restoration, using whatever valve system the department is most familiar with, should be discussed with the patient. Their dexterity, personal hygiene and compliance will need assessing prior to a decision being made about a primary tracheoesophageal puncture. If there is any doubt, defer the decision and consider a secondary puncture months after the laryngectomy.

Antibiotics

These should be commenced on the day of surgery and continued for 5–7 days postoperatively in order to reduce the incidence of both postoperative fistula development and wound infection. A broad-spectrum agent such as augmentin is appropriate.

Incision

A routine apron incision is used, extending from the posterior end of the hyoid on one side down in a U to a point approximately equidistant between the suprasternal notch and the cricoid cartilage, and then back up to the posterior end of the hyoid on the other side. The wound of a pre-existing tracheostomy needs to be excised in its entirety, in continuity with the incision.

If a neck dissection is also being undertaken then the ipsilateral limb of the apron incision can be lateralized by 2–3 cm and extended up to the mastoid process. This is preferable to the alternative option of a lateral limb being taken down to the clavicle, necessitating a three-point junction. If a postoperative salivary fistula develops, this junction will almost certainly break down.

Operative technique

Raise skin flaps

The skin flaps are raised in the subplatysmal plane, and the anterior jugular veins are divided just above the suprasternal notch

Isolation of larynx

A plane of dissection is established along the anterior border of the sternomastoid muscle separating the larynx, thyroid and pharynx from the major vascular compartment of the neck. The omohyoid muscle is defined and divided low in the neck and between clips. The ends of the muscle are diathermized and then released. The sternohyoid muscle and the sternothyroid muscle are managed in the same way. The last three steps are repeated on the other side of the neck (**Figure 7.1**).

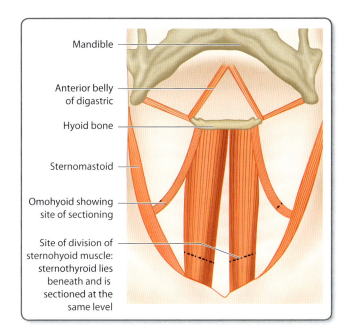

Mandible

Anterior belly
of digastric

Hyoid bone

Sternomastoid

Omohyoid showing
site of sectioning

Site of division of
sternohyoid muscle:
sternothyroid lies
beneath and is
sectioned at the
same level

Figure 7.1 The skin flaps
are raised and the larynx
is mobilized, starting with
division of the anchoring strap
muscles.

- Unless oncologically contraindicated every attempt should be
  made to preserve the thyroid and parathyroid glands on at least
  one side. The thyroid isthmus is defined by sharp dissection
  and then divided between clips. Suture ligate the cut ends of the
  isthmus
- If a lobe is to be preserved, the gland is retracted laterally and is
  separated from the upper trachea and larynx by sharp dissection.
  Diathermy is used to control the inevitable bleeding. This is most
  notable in relation to the ligamentous attachment of the gland
  to larynx at the cricotracheal junction posterolaterally. The lobe
  is now fully mobilized away from the larynx. It should not be
  necessary to disturb the glands arterial supply and venous drainage
  on that side
- If a lobe is to be removed in continuity with the larynx then the
  inferior thyroid vessels, the middle thyroid vein and the superior
  vascular pedicle will all need to be divided and tied. The inferior
  pole of the gland will also require mobilizing off the trachea, up
  to the level of the proposed sectioning of the trachea (**Figure 7.2**).
  The hyoid bone is palpated and the anterior jugular veins are again
  divided where they cross it
- Cutting diathermy is now used to skeletonize the anterior and
  superior surfaces of the bone. Keep directly on the bone in order
  to avoid damage to the lingual arteries or hypoglossal nerves.
  Continue the skeletonization posteriorly and mobilize the greater
  horn of the bone on each side

Divide the superior thyroid pedicle on the side on which the thyroid lobe is being removed, if this has not already been done. Use cutting diathermy to free the inferior pharyngeal constrictor from its attachment to the thyroid cartilage on each side (**Figure 7.3**). On each side use a scalpel to incise the perichondrium of the thyroid cartilage from the tip of the superior cornu right down to the inferior cornu.

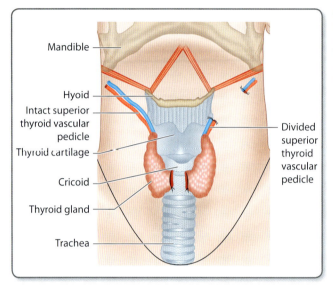

Figure 7.2 As dissection proceeds, the right lobe of the thyroid is mobilized as it is to be preserved. The left lobe is separated from its vascular supply and left attached to the larynx as it is to be resected.

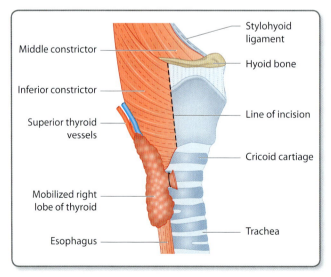

Figure 7.3 Cutting diathermy is used to detach the inferior constrictor from the thyroid cartilage along the incision line illustrated (------). The perichondrium is then incised in the same direction using a knife.

- Mobilize the perichondrium off the cartilage on the side NOT involved by tumor, taking the elevation into the pyriform fossa
- Section the trachea at an appropriate level. Avoid damaging the tracheal ring cartilage immediately inferior. With the close co-operation of the anesthetist, remove the endotracheal tube and place a laryngectomy tube into the newly fashioned stoma
- The sectioning of the trachea can then be completed across its posterior wall. Be careful not to cut right through and button-hole the esophagus. There should be a natural plane of dissection evident between the two structures
- Using individual silk sutures, secure the anterior half of the free edge of the trachea to the lower edge of the skin flap, in the midline. It is quite acceptable to place the suture through the entire tracheal wall immediately below the uppermost ring. Do not try and bisect a cartilaginous tracheal ring with the needle. It is also acceptable to bring the trachea out through a small, separate midline incision some 2 cm below the free edge of the inferior skin flap

Excision of the larynx

- Using cutting diathermy, carefully divide the soft tissues between the tongue base and the larynx, dissecting vertically down toward the posterior pharyngeal wall immediately above the hyoid bone. Do this first on one side if the tumor is known to extend into the vallecula or tongue base on the other. The vallecular mucosa will come into view as will the outline of the epiglottis
- Incise the vallecula mucosa. (It is now important to preserve as much pharyngeal mucosa as possible, without compromising the provision of adequate tumor margins.) Once the larynx has been entered, incise the mucosa along the free edge of the epiglottis on each side (**Figure 7.4**)

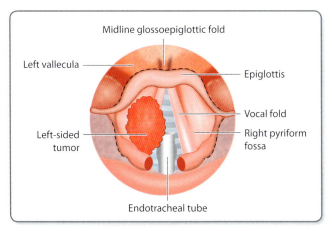

Left vallecula

Midline glossoepiglottic fold

Epiglottis

Vocal fold

Left-sided tumor

Right pyriform fossa

Endotracheal tube

Figure 7.4 The surgeon stands at the head of the operating table and opens the pharynx through the vallecula on the contralateral side to the tumor. The appropriate mucosal incisions can then be made, freeing up the larynx (------). Direct visualization of the tumor is essential.

- At the lower extent of one of these mucosal incisions, develop a submucosal tunnel medially, running across the posterior face of the cricoid cartilage
- With one blade of the scissors in the tunnel and the other in the pharyngeal lumen, divide the mucosal horizontally, thereby connecting up with the mucosal incision of the other side. There should now be no other mucosal attachments between the larynx and pharynx
- Now lift up the larynx, using sharp dissection to free it from the pyriform fossa on each side. (If the tumor involves the aryepiglottic fold and/or the pyriform fossa then the pharynx should not be divided along the lateral edge of the epiglottis but far more laterally, allowing the tumor to be encompassed in continuity with the larynx itself.)
- With a finger in the esophageal lumen dissect the larynx fully away from the pharynx and cervical esophagus without unnecessarily damaging the mucosa of the latter
- The specimen can now be removed and the mucosal margins assessed, using frozen section examination if indicated

Surgical voice restoration

- If a primary tracheoesophageal puncture is being undertaken, retract the upper posterior wall of the trachea superiorly using two Allis forceps applied to the soft tissues immediately adjacent to it. This will put it 'on stretch.' Suture a silk tie onto the tip of a 14F Foley catheter. Introduce a clip into the esophagus via the open pharynx. Maneuver the tip of the clip to tent up the mucosa of the posterior tracheal wall in the midline, about 1 cm below its superior edge (**Figure 7.5**). Using a 2–3 mm incision, cut directly through the mucosa onto the tip of the clip which can then be delivered into the tracheal lumen. The clip is then gently opened, enabling the silk tie and Foley catheter

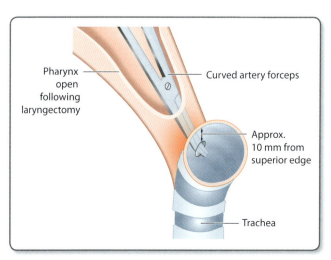

Pharynx open following laryngectomy

Curved artery forceps

Approx. 10 mm from superior edge

Trachea

Figure 7.5 Forceps in the open pharynx 'tent up' the mucosa of the posterior tracheal wall, approximately 1 cm below its free superior edge. A 3 mm horizontal incision is made onto the tip of the instrument, creating a fistula.

to be pulled through from the trachea into the esophagus, thereby establishing the fistula. The suture is then removed, the catheter tip being diverted down into the esophageal lumen. The balloon is inflated with 3–5 mL of air. The catheter can also be used for feeding the patient, negating the requirement of a nasogastric tube
- Closure of the pharynx should be undertaken in two layers using a continuous extramucosal Vicryl followed by interrupted Vicryl sutures to bring the inferior constrictor and tongue base musculature together. A T-shaped closure provides a much better functional result than a straight vertical closure
- Insert a nasogastric tube if a fistula has not been created (**Figure 7.6**)
- Suction drainage is used and the wound closed with Vicryl and then silk, nylon or clips for the skin

Postoperative care

- The drains should be retained for at least 4 days
- If there is no evidence of fistula formation after 1 week in a non-irradiated neck then oral swallowing can commence. In the irradiated neck swallowing should only be allowed after a satisfactory barium swallow undertaken at 10 days. Skin suture removal should follow a similar time course
- In the absence of residual tumor or gross wound breakdown fistulae usually close without the need for surgical intervention. If they persist for >6 weeks then surgical closure should be considered. A pectoralis major flap is usually appropriate.

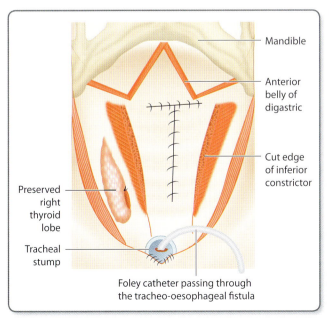

Figure 7.6 T-shaped mucosal closure of the hypopharynx. The inferior constrictors have yet to be sutured together.

Mandible

Anterior belly of digastric

Cut edge of inferior constrictor

Preserved right thyroid lobe

Tracheal stump

Foley catheter passing through the tracheo-oesophageal fistula

Gastrostomy feeding should be considered in patients with significant long-term fistulae
- Once oral swallowing has resumed the tracheoesophageal catheter can be replaced by a speech valve. If the patient has not been punctured then the development of esophageal speech or the use of a Servox-type vibrator should be considered
- Stomal stenosis rarely develops after surgery and may require the use of a stoma button or laryngectomy tube. If it persists long term, in the absence of local infection or tumor recurrence, then surgery should be considered although results can be disappointing

Further reading

Shah JP, Patel S, Singh B (eds). Jatin Shah's Head and Neck Surgery and Oncology, 4th edn. Philadelphia, PA: Mosby Elsevier, 2012.

Tonsil and soft palate surgery

Stephen Crank

The tonsil, soft palate and tongue base (Chapter 9) are the important anatomical subsites of the oropharynx. The tonsil is the main component of the lateral oropharyngeal wall which extends from the palatoglossal arch (anterior pillar) to palatopharyngeal arch (posterior pillar). In continuity with the lateral oropharyngeal wall is the retromolar region of the oral cavity anteriorly and the posterior wall of the oropharynx posteriorly.

The soft palate is the roof of the oropharynx that is a mobile muscular flap that extends from the posterior aspect of the hard palate and separates the nasopharynx from the oropharynx. The oral surface of the soft palate is in the oropharynx and extends laterally on each side to the lateral pharyngeal wall and tonsillar regions. The lateral aspect of the oropharynx is in continuity with the parapharyngeal space.

Squamous cell carcinoma's are the most frequent malignancy and account for 90% of oropharyngeal tumors. Traditionally, oropharyngeal SCC has been related to tobacco and alcohol habits but the important role of HPV is now recognized. Other neoplasms of the oropharynx include lymphoma arising from lymphoid tissue and salivary gland tumors, both benign and malignant, from the minor salivary glands.

Assessment and diagnosis of oropharyngeal tumors

Oropharyngeal tumors can present in a variety of ways including soreness of the throat, otalgia, dysphagia, ulceration, or the feeling of a lump. Patients who present with trismus often have extensive disease with infiltration and resulting fixity of the medial pterygoid muscle or further extension of the lesion and mandibular invasion. The presence of a neck mass is indicative of regional metastatic disease.

Evaluation of patients with oropharyngeal malignancy requires an accurate history and examination with flexible nasendoscopy and palpation of region. Cross-sectional imaging with MRI evaluates the soft tissue in the oropharyngeal region (**Figures 8.1** and **8.2**) and may be supplemented by USS to further assess the neck. The role of PET–CT is evolving but is useful in the demonstration of occult oropharyngeal primaries presenting with neck metastases.

Definitive diagnosis requires histological confirmation and a formal examination under general anesthesia with panendoscopy and associated biopsy is essential. In a small number of cases, it may be possible under local anesthesia to biopsy an anterior lesion of the soft palate or palatoglossal fold. Biopsies are usually performed taking an ellipse of abnormal tissue which includes the margin of the lesion. For the tonsil, a decision needs to be made whether an incisional biopsy is performed or more preferably a standard tonsillectomy.

Treatment options for soft palate and tonsil tumors

The decision as to the management of soft palate and tonsil tumors will depend upon:
- Pathology – benign or malignant
- Size of tumor
- Location of tumor

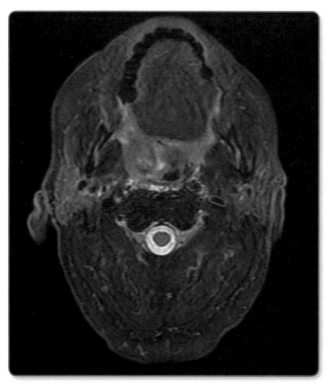

Figure 8.1 Axial MRI scan of patient with a recurrent SCC of the right oropharynx following treatment with radical chemoradiotherapy. This patient was treated with salvage surgery with a lip split and mandibulotomy with resection and reconstruction with a radial forearm free flap.

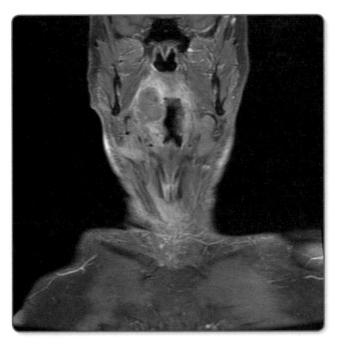

Figure 8.2 Coronal MRI scan of the same patient as Figure 8.1. The two views allow the full extent of the tumour to be visualised allowing careful surgical planning with respect to the resection and required margins.

- Neck status – node positive or negative
- Previous treatment – in particular, previous radiotherapy
- Requirement of reconstruction and likely functional outcome
- Need for an access procedure

Currently, it is generally accepted that chemoradiotherapy is the primary modality of treatment for most cases of squamous cell carcinoma of the tonsil and soft palate. However, surgery is indicated in specific cases.

Soft palate surgery

Soft palate surgery can often be performed via a per-oral approach utilizing either a gag or mouth prop. The main indications for surgery to treat soft palate neoplasms include:

- Benign disease
- Malignant disease which is radiation resistant, e.g. salivary gland malignancy including adenoid cystic carcinoma, mucoepidermoid carcinomas
- Small localized T1 lesions that can be easily excised and defect closed
- Recurrent disease following failure of radiotherapy

The site and size of the lesion within the soft palate is important in planning the surgical management and reconstruction:

- Small lesions of the posterior aspect and free margin of the soft palate are amenable to resection with an appropriate margin and primary closure. The prime illustration of this type of lesion is a small carcinoma of the uvula which can be readily removed safely via a per-oral approach with associated primary closure

- Lesions of the central region of the soft palate can be readily resected by a per-oral approach. This is particularly relevant for benign disease of the minor salivary glands such as a pleomorphic adenoma. An appropriate oncological margin is still required and this often necessitates a full-thickness soft palate resection. Providing the posterior free margin of the soft palate has not been removed then usually the defect can be repaired with a rotation flap from the hard palate based on the greater palatine vessels. This flap is raised in the subperiosteal plane and rotated to repair the defect. A dressing plate is fabricated to cover the exposed bone of the hard palate, this may be secured with clasps to the teeth or screwed into the hard palate, and a dressing (e.g. zinc oxide/eugenol) is placed beneath the plate. The plate is left for 3 weeks to allow the palate to granulate and epithelialize (**Figure 8.3**)
- Lesions which are more extensive, extend from the soft palate into the tonsil or palatoglossal fold and tongue base, or involve a significant length of the soft palate and breach the posterior margin require an access procedure to fully visualize and permit a safe oncological resection. The preferred access procedure is a lip split mandibulotomy procedure which is described later. With the removal of larger volumes of soft palate tissue there is the need to reconstruct the soft palate with either a regional flap such as a temporalis muscle flap or a free flap such as the radial forearm flap

Complications

- Breakdown of flaps and wounds result in the development of an oronasal fistula. Regurgitation of fluids and food through the fistula can be upsetting and distressing to patients and a cause of social embarrassment. Most small fistulae resolve with the use of a cover plate extending over the fistula to prevent reflux and allow healing of the fistula. In some patients, the cover plate may be difficult to wear if extended too far posteriorly, resulting in a significant gag reflex. When a large fistula has reduced in size it can usually be closed with excision of the fistula and a small flap repair, e.g. rhomboid flap, or simply left to close by secondary intention. In cases of persistent large fistulae that do not respond to conservative treatment a formal reconstruction may be indicated
- Velopharyngeal incompetence with the development of hypernasal speech, and regurgitation of fluids due to contracture and shortening of the soft palate. This requires input from a speech and language therapists to fully evaluate palatal function. Further reconstruction or a pharyngoplasty may be required to decrease the incompetence
- Difficulty swallowing following the reconstruction of large soft palate defects using insensate skin flaps results in an inability to control the movement of the food bolus. Speech and language

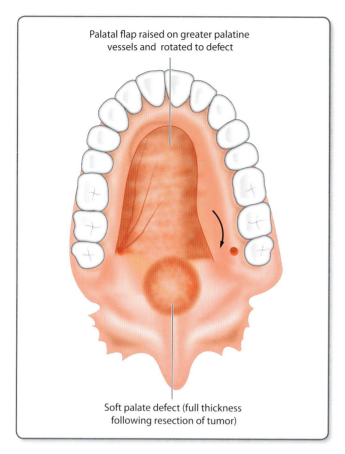

Palatal flap raised on greater palatine
vessels and rotated to defect

Soft palate defect (full thickness
following resection of tumor)

Figure 8.3 Palatal rotation flap to repair a defect created following full thickness resection of a small midline and anterior soft palate tumour in which the posterior margin of the soft palate is maintained. The palatal rotation flap is a full thickness mucoperiosteal flap and the donor site covered with a dressing plate and allowed to heal.

therapy input is required and in extreme cases patients may be dependent on a long-term feeding tube in order to avoid aspiration

Tonsil and lateral oropharyngeal wall surgery

The tonsil is usually removed in its entirety in the assessment and diagnosis of malignancy at this site. For small lesions this may provide a complete excision and oncological clearance of the tumor. When clinical or radiological examination suggests a large primary malignancy an incisional biopsy is usually performed.

The indications for surgical management of tonsillar and lateral oropharyngeal wall malignancy are similar to those indications for definitive soft palate surgery and include salvage surgery for recurrent or radioresistant disease, salivary gland malignancy or extensive disease that has spread anteriorly to the retromolar region and involved mandibular bone. To adequately resect a tonsil and lateral oropharyngeal wall tumor an access procedure is required for which the lip split mandibulotomy is the preferred procedure.

Lip split mandibulotomy approach to the oropharynx

The lip split mandibulotomy approach is essential in accessing and permitting a safe oncological resection of many lesions of the oropharynx. If a lesion cannot be safely removed by a per-oral approach then the lip split mandibulotomy approach should be utilized. It is also used to access the parapharyngeal space lateral to the lateral wall of the oropharynx. The technique also provides access to allow reconstruction of the oropharynx and facilitates the placement and inset of flaps.

There are variations at differing stages of the technique but essentially the procedure involves an incision to divide the lower lip and chin, an osteotomy of the mandible in the symphyseal or parasymphyseal region and release of the tissues in the floor of mouth and submandibular region.

Preoperative assessment is essential. Along with standard scanning and a chest X-ray, an orthopantomogram, is taken to image the mandible. A lip spilt mandibulotomy is usually undertaken in conjunction with a neck dissection.

Operative technique

- The incision for the neck dissection is extended up to the submental region which will later permit extension of this incision into the chin and the lip
- Subplatysmal flaps are raised in the neck to the lower border of the mandible. The marginal mandibular branch of the facial nerve is dissected out and protected, the facial vessels divided and the periosteum of the mandible incised and following this the neck dissection proceeds and is completed as required
- The neck incision is extended from the submental region up through the chin and the lip – the preference is for the incision to be placed into the labiomental groove around the chin button, either as a curve following the chin button or as multiple small 'Zs' which is aesthetically pleasing due to a scar within the natural facial lines (Hayter et al. 1996). Other options do exist which include a straight vertical cut or a Z directly across the chin button (**Figure 8.4**)
- The incision is continued through the vermillion of the lip with diathermy or ligation of the labial arteries
- The incision is completed through the full thickness of the lip with incision of the intra oral labial mucosa and then extended onto the gingivae of the lower anterior teeth and includes a complete interdental papilla. There is further planned release with the incision placed in the gingival crevice incising the periodontal fibers of the teeth to permit the mucoperiosteal flaps to be raised. All incisions onto the mandible fully incise the periosteum
- Using a Freers or Howarths periosteal elevator a subperiosteal dissection is performed to expose the mandible and then identify and expose the mental nerve on the side of which the osteotomy is planned

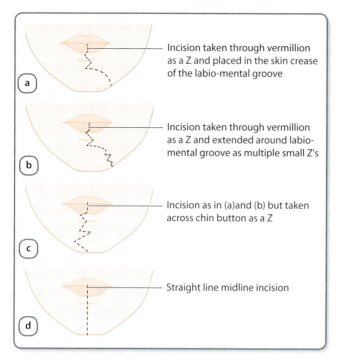

Incision taken through vermillion as a Z and placed in the skin crease of the labio-mental groove

Incision taken through vermillion as a Z and extended around labio-mental groove as multiple small Z's

Incision as in (a) and (b) but taken across chin button as a Z

Straight line midline incision

Figure 8.4 Possible options for the incision of the lip split through the chin point. The preferred options are (a) and (b) which give a good aesthetic result, hiding the incision in the labiomental groove and breaking up the incision with multiple Zs through the lip. Option (c) comes across the chin button as a Z which can also give a pleasing aesthetic result. Option (d) is least preferable with an obvious scar and least pleasing aesthetic result.

- Mandibular plates are adapted to the mandible (2.0 mm plates, at least four-hole spaced) at the site of the planned osteotomy and all holes drilled and plates secured prior to being removed
- The lingual mucoperiosteum is incised and released at the site of the osteotomy
- A stepped osteotomy is performed in the parasymphyseal region avoiding the tooth roots. A fine reciprocating saw is used to make the cut through the buccal and lingual cortex and the osteotomy completed with fine osteotomes and the mandible split (**Figure 8.5**)
- Following completion of the osteotomy, the floor of mouth and submandibular tissues need to be fully released to allow the mandible to be swung laterally and 'open the door' to provide the required access
- The floor of mouth mucosa is incised lateral to the submandibular duct leaving a good cuff of lingual mucosa to allow closure at the end of the procedure. It is essential to divide mylohyoid in the neck to free the mandible but adequate muscle should be left to allow the muscle to be closed
- The floor of mouth incision is taken posteriorly to the oropharyngeal region but it is essential that tumor is not encroached upon
- These steps should permit adequate access to the tumor visualizing the full extent of the lesion and in particular it's inferior and posterior extent
- Appropriate excision of the primary tumor can now be undertaken, with an appropriate margin of normal mucosa and soft tissue to

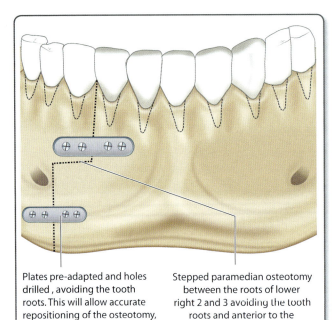

Figure 8.5 Stepped osteotomy in the paramedian region. The cuts are made between the roots of the teeth avoiding damage to the roots and also considering the mental nerve. Plates are pre-adapted and holes drilled permitting accurate realignment and re-establishment of the dental occlusion.

Plates pre-adapted and holes drilled , avoiding the tooth roots. This will allow accurate repositioning of the osteotomy, re-establishing the dental occlusion.

Stepped paramedian osteotomy between the roots of lower right 2 and 3 avoiding the tooth roots and anterior to the mental nerve.

obtain adequate clearance. Frozen section analysis of margins should be used as necessary

Closure

Once the tumor has been resected and a flap, if required, inset into the lip split, the mandibulotomy is closed. Firstly, the oral mucosa is realigned and closed with a 3-0 resorbable suture and if adequate cuffs of mucosa have been left this should be performed with ease. The osteotomy is replaced and realigned with the preadapted plates to re-establish the correct dental occlusion. Meticulous attention is directed to a layered closure of the skin including accurate repositioning of the skin and vermillion border.

Postoperative care

Once it is deemed that healing of the surgical site and flap has occurred and diet reintroduced after 7–10 days postsurgery, care must still be taken with eating and chewing for 6 weeks while bone healing at the osteotomy site proceeds. Postoperative X-rays (Orthopantomograph and PA Mandible) should be taken for records and to ensure accurate realignment of the osteotomy.

Complications of lip split mandibulotomy

- Numbness to the lower lip – this occurs due to trauma to the mental nerve. The nerve is identified and protected at the time the osteotomy is performed and therefore any resultant paraethesia or anesthesia to the lower lip should be transient due to a neuropraxia

- Numbness to the tongue is due to lingual nerve injury resulting from the floor of mouth incision as it is extended posteriorly. It should be avoidable
- Damage to the roots of the teeth – this may occur due to the vertical cuts between the tooth roots or the horizontal cuts being placed incorrectly at the level of the tooth roots. If the teeth become non-vital they may need to be root filled or removed
- Malocclusion postoperatively – this should be prevented by careful surgery both prior to the osteotomy, when the plates are adapted to the mandible, and by careful realignment and fixation of the mandible when the osteotomy is plated
- Non-union or delayed union, this may be associated with metalwork failure and may require the use of heavier plates and fixation. The other main reason would be the osteotomy being performed in a previously irradiated field, something which should be avoided if at all possible
- Poor aesthetic result due to the lip split – this can be prevented with the careful placement of incisions in skin crease lines and the careful realignment of wounds particularly at the vermillion border of the lip
- Breakdown of the floor of mouth and fistula formation, this may be as a result of not maintaining an adequate cuff of tissue to reapproximate and close when the floor of mouth incision is made

T4 lateral oropharyngeal tumors involving mandibular bone

In cases of extensive tonsillar carcinoma there maybe direct invasion of the tumor into the mandibular bone. This may occur with the tumor extending anteriorly to the retromolar region of the mandible or spread through the medial pterygoid muscle to the medial cortex of the mandibular ramus. In addition to clinical examination including the assessment of trismus, mandibular invasion is evaluated through plain X-ray, CT (looking specifically at cortical bone involvement) and MR (assessing marrow involvement). If removal of mandibular bone is required to obtain a margin in the resection of a tumor in close proximity to the mandible, but mandibular invasion has not been demonstrated, then a rim or marginal mandibular resection is indicated. For a carcinoma that is shown to invade the mandible then a segmental mandibular resection must be performed.

If a segmental mandibular resection is required then this must be carefully planned with regards to access and volume of bone to be resected. Rather than utilizing a lip split and mandibulotomy with a mandibular swing for access, a more lateral approach is employed.

- Subplatysmal skin flaps are raised in the neck: usually, a neck dissection is required either for oncological reasons or to provide vessel access for the reconstruction. The flaps are raised up to the mandible protecting the marginal mandibular branch of VII and the periosteum of the lower border of the mandible is incised

- A decision will need to be made whether a lip split is required for access (lip split only; not with a mandibulotomy).If required then the incision from the neck is extended as described above to extend only through the lip. Otherwise, the resection is performed via a combination of a per-oral and neck approach

- Using monopolar diathermy, the appropriate margin in the soft tissues lateral to the mandible are incised and then deepened through to the mandibular periosteum. This should provide a good cuff of lateral mandibular soft tissue for oncological clearance and may include masseter

- A periosteal elevator is used via an intra- and extraoral approach to strip soft tissue off the mandible at the site of the proposed osteotomy. Subperiosteal stripping is performed away from the lateral cuff of tissue attached to the mandible. This will expose the mandibular body anterior to the tumor. It is also vital to strip periosteum posterior to the tumor to the posterior border of the mandible and sigmoid notch

- The initial anterior osteotomy cut is made with a reciprocating saw. This is placed in the mandibular body region between the lower first molar and canine depending on the extent of the tumor. The saw cut is made via the neck incision and completed with fine spatula osteotomes

- The condylar head is very rarely involved and can usually be left rather than resected. Therefore, the posterior osteotomy cut is made from the sigmoid notch to the posterior border of the mandibular ramus. This will leave approximately a 1–2 cm fragment of condylar head and neck in situ. Langenbeck retractors are used to retract the soft tissues and the osteotomy cut is made with a saw and completed with osteotomes. If for oncological reasons the condylar head needs to be resected then it is best approached by a modified preauricular incision (Bramley & Al-Kyatt 1979). The insertion of the lateral pterygoid muscle into the fovea of the condylar head needs to be divided and the articular disc of the joint released to allow mobilization and disarticulation of the condyle

- The free segment of mandible is now retraced inferiorly into the neck. It is now essential to fully free the mandible by releasing the temporalis attachment to the coronoid process. This is performed with monopolar diathermy and the mandible can be felt to 'give' when the attachment is fully released

- The tumor can now be resected by mobilizing the specimen into the neck and releasing the tissues medial to the mandible, visualizing the tumor and performing a safe oncological resection. However, care does need to be taken with regards to the major vessels and it is prudent to dissect out, skeletonize and protect these vessels prior to completing the resection

Reconstruction

Reconstruction is essential to close the defect and provide a watertight seal to prevent fistulation. If bone is resected then ideally it should be replaced. A composite free fibula flap provides good length of bone that can be osteotomized to replace body and ramus segments. In addition, the skin paddle of the fibula flap replaces the soft-tissue lining of the oropharynx. For patients who are medically compromised or in patients undergoing salvage surgery with a vessel depleted neck a pedicled pectoralis major or latissimus dorsi myocutaneous flap may be preferable.

Summary

Surgery for tonsil and soft palate tumors can be performed for both diagnostic and treatment purposes. The evolution of chemoradiation has reduced the need for major respective procedures, although surgery is still indicated for smaller lesions of the soft palate, benign and radioresistant lesions, primary cases with mandibular involvement and the salvage case. For access, the need for a lip split mandibulotomy procedure is essential to allow an oncological safe resection for larger soft palate, tonsil, lateral wall lesions and parapharyngeal lesions.

Further reading

Evans B, Lang D. Access surgery. In: Langdon J, Patel M, Ord R, Brennan P (eds), Operative oral and maxillofacial surgery, 2nd edn. London: Hodder Arnold, 2011.

Ward Booth P, Schendel S, Hausamen J-A (eds). Ablative surgical treatment for malignant tumours of the oral cavity. In: Maxillofacial surgery, 2nd edn. London: Churchill Livingstone 2006, pp 419 -439.

References

Bramley P, Al-Kayatt A. A modified pre-auricular approach to the temporo-mandibular joint and malar arch. Br J Oral Surg 1979; 17:91–103.

Hayter JP, Vaughan ED, Brown JS. Aesthetic lip splits. Br J Oral Maxillofac Surg 1996; 35:432–5.

Tongue base surgery

Stephen Crank

The tongue base, or pharyngeal tongue, extends from the circumvallate papillae anteriorly to the vallecula and pre-epiglottic space postero-inferiorly.

Tongue base tumors may remain asymptomatic until they reach an advanced stage, and are frequently diagnosed in the investigation of patients presenting with metastatic neck disease from a perceived occult primary malignancy. Due to the advanced stage of presentation these tumors often cross the midline and directly invade into neighboring structures. They may extend forward into the oral tongue, posteriorly and inferiorly toward the supraglottis and glottis, and laterally to the lower pole of the tonsil and lateral pharyngeal wall.

Squamous cell carcinomas arising from the mucosa of the tongue base are the most common malignancy at this site. Other tongue base lesions include benign and malignant salivary gland tumors originating from the minor salivary glands and lymphomas arising from the lymphoid tissue of Waldeyer's ring at this site.

Surgery, which can be challenging due to the limited access afforded by the per-oral route, has a role in both the diagnosis and definitive surgical management of neoplasms at this site.

Diagnostic surgery for tongue base lesions

The diagnosis of tongue base lesions requires a detailed history and examination including digital palpation of the tongue base and flexible nasendoscopy, supplemented with cross-sectional imaging of which MRI is the preferred modality to fully evaluate the soft tissues. A biopsy is essential for definitive diagnosis. Tissue is usually obtained in conjunction with a formal examination under general anesthesia allowing full clinical evaluation of the tumor. The methods for tissue biopsy include the following:

- The use of biopsy forceps through a pharyngoscope when obvious mucosal disease is present
- If there is a need to obtain deep or submucosal tissue at the tongue base a direct approach is utilized. Maximum mouth opening is obtained through the use of a gag or mouth prop, traction sutures, 2.0 black silk, are placed into the substance of the anterior tongue and used to advance the tongue as far as possible out of the mouth. An incision is made as close as possible to the palpable mass on the posterior dorsum of the tongue that will open the tongue to permit access into deeper tissues. Usually the tumor is evident once these deep tissues are opened and an adequate-sized biopsy can be taken. Hemostasis is achieved with bipolar diathermy and the incision closed with 3.0 resorbable sutures. Alternatively, a tru-cut biopsy needle can be employed for deeply seated tumors

Surgical resection of tongue base tumors

If considering resection of a tongue base tumor then adequate access must be obtained to visualize the lesion and permit completion of a safe and oncologically sound resection. Compromising this fundamental principle will result in a higher than desired incidence of involved or close margins and ultimate failure of treatment.

For squamous cell carcinoma of the tongue base, primary chemoradiotherapy is currently accepted as the preferred modality of treatment. Chemoradiotherapy negates the requirement of complex head and neck surgery including an access osteotomy and resection of large volumes of tongue base tissue requiring free flap reconstruction. The survival rates for both modalities of treatment – surgery and chemo-radiotherapy – are comparable but the great advantage of the latter is that preservation of function in terms of swallowing and speech is far more likely. Patients with human papillomavirus (HPV)-related squamous carcinoma are particularly susceptible to chemoradiotherapy.

There still remain specific indications for ablative surgery for tongue base lesions, namely:

- Salvage procedures where chemoradiotherapy has failed, recurrent disease is deemed resectable and there is no evidence of distant metastases on imaging (usually CT or PET-CT)
- Benign disease, e.g. benign salivary gland tumors
- Radioresistant malignant disease, e.g. salivary gland malignancies such as mucoepidermoid carcinoma, adenoid cystic carcinoma
- Small lesions that can be easily cleared by a per-oral approach without complex reconstruction

Careful consideration is required when planning the most appropriate approach for the treatment of tongue base lesions. The principle of the need of adequate access must always be adhered to and therefore the following options exist:

- A per-oral approach, as described above for the open biopsy of deep tongue base lesions, may be suitable to resect small lesions that can be visualized and removed safely. These sites can be closed primarily or left to heal by secondary intention. The per-oral approach may be undertaken with standard surgical instruments or with a carbon dioxide laser. However, such cases are rare
- Access procedures to open up this surgical site to facilitate an oncologically safe surgical resection

Possible access procedures include a lip split and mandibulotomy, visor neck approach with chin-point osteotomy and drop down, or a pharyngotomy approach through the neck and lateral wall of the pharynx to the tongue base

To determine the optimum approach depends upon consideration of a number of factors which include the laterality and exact site of the tumor, requirement of a neck dissection, if any, or neck access for reconstruction, and the reconstructive needs of the patient and cosmetic considerations. This is detailed in **Figure 9.1**. In addition, the patient's overall medical status needs to be fully evaluated and optimized for those undergoing this form of major head and neck surgery.

The lip split and mandibulotomy approach is flexible, straight-forward to perform and provides good access to the tongue base and oropharynx. It is described in Chapter 8. However, the visor approach with a chin-point osteotomy (Merrick et al. 2007) does have some advantages over the lip split/mandibulotomy approach for tongue base access. These include the following:

- The mandible is kept in continuity with a box osteotomy of vascularized bone of the chin point. This is important in patients who have been irradiated, preventing any complications of non-union or delayed union of the mandible. In addition, there would be no likelihood of occlusal discrepancy following reduction and fixation of the osteotomy
- No further incisions are required if performed in conjunction with a bilateral neck dissection which is often required to manage the neck in tongue base lesions
- The cosmetic outcome as there is no lip splitting incision
- Excellent access is obtained

The only contraindication to this approach is a thin edentulous mandible where it would not be possible to perform a chin-point osteotomy and leave a significant height of mandible intact with adequate inherent strength to avoid the risk of fracture.

Operative technique of visor approach with chin-point osteotomy

- A visor incision is utilized extending from mastoid-to-mastoid in a mid-cervical skin crease of the neck. The skin flaps are raised in the subplatysmal plane towards the lower border of the mandible, the marginal mandibular branch of the facial nerve is identified and dissected out on each side, raised superiorly and protected

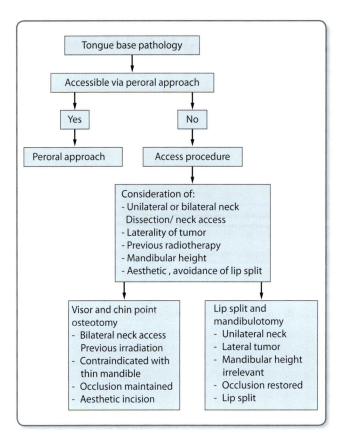

Figure 9.1 Algorithm detailing the decision-making for surgical management of tongue base pathology.

- The lower border of the mandible is exposed in the subperiosteal plane from mandibular angle-to-mandibular angle, dividing and ligating the facial vessels on each side
- If required neck dissections are performed bilaterally or unilaterally. At a minimum Level I must be cleared bilaterally to allow exposure of mylohyoid for successful completion of the approach
- The periosteum is further stripped and reflected in the midline of the mandible to fully expose the chin point of the mandible. The mental foramina are identified bilaterally and the mental nerves protected
- A marking pen is used to outline the proposed box osteotomy of the chin point, this osteotomy consists of a horizontal limb which must be placed above the genial tubercles and two lateral limbs on either side anterior to the mental nerves
- Titanium mini plates (2.0 mm plates) are adapted across the proposed osteotomy site, holes drilled and 6 mm screws placed. Following this the plates are removed and stored safely to be replaced later

- The chin-point osteotomy is performed with a fine blade reciprocating saw. The cut is deepened through the full depth of the mandible and then the cut completed with fine osteotomes. This chin-point is now free but pedicled on the anterior belly of digastric, genioglossus and geniohyoid muscles (**Figure 9.2**)
- The mylohyoid is divided bilaterally with cutting diathermy in the horizontal plane. This division is made at the mid-point of the muscle so when the wounds closed the muscle can be sutured together with ease rather than attempting to suture the muscle to its hyoid or mandibular attachment. Division of the muscle will allow the floor of mouth, when released, to be 'dropped down' into the neck
- The oral cavity is entered. An incision needs to be made to release the lingual mucoperiosteum from retromolar to retromolar region. For a dentate patient it is preferred if this is a crevicular incision with a No. 15 blade down the periodontal membrane of the standing teeth. For an edentulous patient then this can be a crestal incision over the edentulous ridge. Following this the lingual mucoperiosteum is released from the lingual aspect of the mandible with a Freers or Howarths elevator. It is necessary to release the mylohyoid attachment over the mylohyoid ridge (**Figure 9.3**)
- It should now be possible to drop the tongue including the base of tongue into the neck. This will provide good access to resect the tumor. Traction sutures (2-0 silk) are placed into the anterior tongue away from the tumor. Langenbeck retractors are placed under the mandibular body and the mandible retracted superiorly

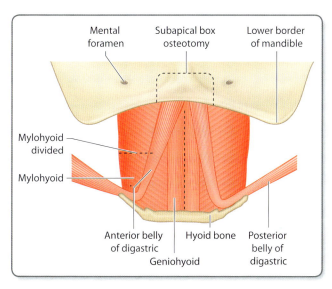

Figure 9.2 Schematic diagram of the initial stages of a chin-point osteotomy and pull through approach. Via a visor incision, the skin flaps are raised and the mandible is exposed. An osteotomy is performed beneath the roots of the lower anterior teeth anterior to the mental foramina and incorporating the anterior belly of digastric and genial tubercles.

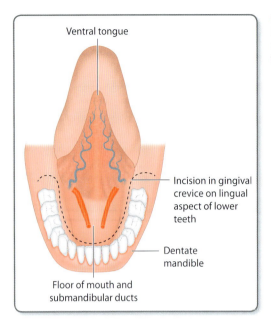

Ventral tongue

Incision in gingival
crevice on lingual
aspect of lower
teeth

Dentate
mandible

Floor of mouth and
submandibular ducts

Figure 9.3 The floor of mouth is released via an incision in the lingual gingival crevice or on the crest in edentulous patients. This allows the tongue and floor of mouth to be pulled through into the neck.

while the tongue, attached to the chin-point osteotomy is pulled down into the neck via the traction sutures (**Figure 9.4**)
- Resection of the tumor can now proceed safely with good visualization and palpation of the lesion. The reconstruction can also proceed while access is obtained

Closure
- After resection of the tumor, and reconstruction of the defect as required, the osteotomy is closed. Initially, the lingual mucoperiosteum is closed with a resorbable 3-0 or 4-0 suture either directly or with vertical mattress sutures around the necks of the teeth
- The chin-point osteotomy is then realigned, the previously adapted mini plates are applied and the osteotomy secured with screws in the predrilled holes
- Mylohyoid is then sutured with a continuous resorbable suture
- Drains are placed and the neck closed in layers with clips to the skin

Possible complications

1. Damage to tooth roots in the lower labial segment is possible when the osteotomy cuts are made and completed. The teeth could be apiceted or rendered non-vital requiring root canal treatment. It is essential that adequate preoperative radiography in the form of an orthopantomogram is undertaken to accurately assess the length and morphology of all roots
2. Non-union of the osteotomy site is possible but unlikely as the chin-point osteotomy is a vascularized segment of bone based on

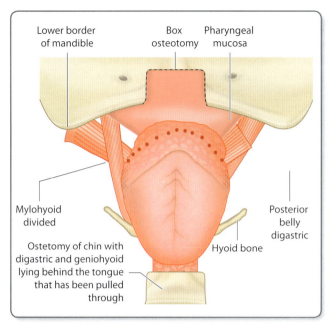

Lower border of mandible

Box osteotomy

Pharyngeal mucosa

Mylohyoid divided

Posterior belly digastric

Ostetomy of chin with digastric and geniohyoid lying behind the tongue that has been pulled through

Hyoid bone

Figure 9.4 The tongue is pulled through into the neck allowing good access to the tongue base and an oncologically safe resection. The chin-point osteotomy is pedicled on the anterior belly of digastric and geniohyoid.

the digastric muscles and there are no significant occlusal forces on the segment. If it does occur, it is usually because the mandible has been previously irradiated
3. Damage to nerves with resultant weakness of the lower lip as a consequence of facial nerve injury and damage to the mental nerves with numbness or altered sensation of the lower lips. Both of these injuries should be temporary and neurapraxic in nature

Lateral pharyngotomy approach to the tongue base

Although the lateral pharyngotomy approach can be used to access tongue base lesions, visualization of the tumor can still be suboptimal, particularly if there is significant medial extent of the tumor, resulting in a compromised tumor resection. Usually, the lateral pharyngotomy approach is performed in conjunction with a neck dissection and utilizes the neck dissection approach. Otherwise, a cervical skin crease incision is used at the level of the hyoid to access the neck. Dissection to the lateral pharynx then continues medial to the carotid sheath. The suprahyoid muscles are divided from the lateral aspect of the hyoid bone to expose the pharyngeal wall. The pharynx is then opened at the level of the vallecula using scissors and Langenbeck retractors inserted to retract the pharyngeal wall mucosa for access and visualization of the tumor.

The tumor can then be removed by sharp dissection or CO_2 laser. It is advisable to routinely use frozen section analysis of margins in all tongue base resections.

Reconstruction of tongue base defects

The aims of reconstruction of the tongue base are to optimize postoperative function, namely speech and swallowing, and to provide a watertight seal to prevent development of a salivary fistula. It is imperative that movement of the tongue is maintained and scarring and narrowing of the oropharynx prevented. For small defects primary closure is possible but larger defects will require a flap reconstruction. The radial forearm free flap provides thin and pliable tissue to maintain tongue movement and function. If greater bulk is required and the resection extends significantly into the anterior two thirds of the tongue, the anterolateral thigh or free rectus flap will provide greater volume of tissue. Other possible options for reconstruction include the pedicled pectoralis major flap which can provide a large volume of tissue and can be of use in the salvage case and vessel depleted neck.

For the larger soft tissue tongue base defects, long-term swallowing may remain difficult and the input of a speech and language therapist is imperative. Long-term nutritional support through a feeding gastrostomy often required. If combined modality treatment is required, i.e. surgery and postoperative radiotherapy then functional outcomes are likely to be poor.

If both hypoglossal nerves are damaged or resected then the patient suffers what are effectively the same consequences that follow a total glossectomy. This should always be avoided if at all possible.

Future developments

The development of robotic surgery permits improved visualization of tongue base pathology with the associated safer resection of tongue base defects without the need for an access procedure. This area of head and neck surgery for the treatment of oropharyngeal disease will increase in the future as such technology becomes more accessible.

Summary

Tongue base surgery can be challenging due to the requirement to obtain adequate access to enable a safe oncological approach for clearance of tumors at this site. The lip split and mandibulotomy approach and the visor approach with chin-point osteotomy are the preferred methods of obtaining access to this difficult site. However, the visor and chin-point osteotomy approach with a pull down does have advantages over other approaches in respect of access, healing and possible decreased postoperative complications.

Further reading

Shah JP, Patel S, Singh B (eds). Jatin Shah's Head and Neck Surgery and Oncology, 4th edn. Philadelphia, PA: Mosby Elsevier, 2012.

Watkinson JC, Gilbert RW (eds). Stell and Maran's Head and Neck Surgery, 4th edn. London: Hodder Arnold, 2012.

References

Merrick GD, Morrison RW, Gallagher JR, Devine JC. Pedicled genial osteotomy modification of the mandibular release operation for access to the back of the tongue. Br J Oral Maxillofacial Surg 2007; 45:490–92.

Medial maxillectomy via a lateral rhinotomy approach

John Waldron

A medical maxillectomy involves removal of the lateral nasal wall and ethmoid air cells up to the level of the cribriform plate superiorly and to the pterygoid plates posteriorly.

The classical approach to a medial maxillectomy utilizes the lateral rhinotomy incision. It is possible to perform a partial medial maxillectomy via a mid-facial degloving approach. It is difficult to reach the upper part of the ethmoid air cells through this incision. Improvements in endoscopic techniques now allow a proportion of tumors previously approached through a lateral rhinotomy incision to be resected endoscopically without the need for an external skin incision.

Preoperative considerations

- The tumor type should be confirmed histologically by a biopsy prior to the resection. This can normally be accomplished in the outpatient setting using local topical anesthetic if necessary
- The tumor extent is visualized endoscopically and the patient should also have CT scanning which is particularly useful for looking at bony destruction. An MRI may also be needed to help differentiate the soft tissue extent of the tumor from retained secretions in the sinuses
- If the histology shows a tumor type with the risk of metastatic spread to the chest, abdomen, or pelvis, then CT scans of these areas should also be performed prior to surgery. An alternative is a PET-CT scan

Surgical anatomy

The key anatomical features are shown in **Figure 10.1** and the extent of bone removal with necessary osteotomies in **Figure 10.2**.

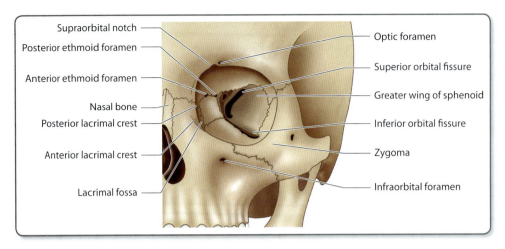

Figure 10.1 Bony anatomy.

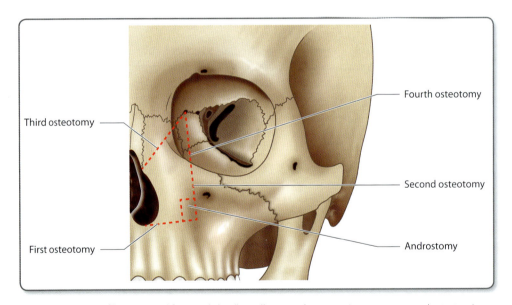

Figure 10.2 Extent of bone removal for a medial wall maxillectomy, demonstrating antrostomy and osteotomies.

Consent

The nature of the resulting scar should be explained to patients. along with the risks of possible visual loss or diplopia are discussed. They should be told that they may also suffer from epiphora and from crusting or bleeding in the nasal cavity. It is also important to explain the potential for a CSF leak or meningitis which can happen after this surgery.

If the tumor has metastized to the neck it may also be necessary to consider a neck dissection.

The operation

The operation is normally carried out under a general anesthetic using endotracheal intubation. It is not necessary to have prophylactic antibiotic cover for this surgery.

Incision

The incision is shown in **Figure 10.3**. The incision passes through a point midway between the midline and the medial canthus. The incision passes down the lateral wall of the nose and extends around and 2–3 mm lateral to the alar crease into the nostril. It is useful to tattoo a few points with methylene blue prior to making the incision to allow maximum precision of the closure.

A tarsorrhaphy is performed using a fine silk suture to prevent any damage to the cornea during surgery.

The incision line is infiltrated with a mixture of 2% Xylocaine and 1 in 80,000 Epinephrine to reduce bleeding from the skin edges.

The nasal cavity on that side is filled with a decongestant solution which is left for 10 minutes prior to surgery being started. This is then removed using aspiration.

Operative technique

A blade is used to incise down onto and through the periosteum in the line of the incision. Hemostasis is obtained using bipolar cautery. The major bleeding that occurs is from the angular vessels which are usually transected near the medial canthus. Bleeding from these can be controlled with either bipolar cautery or by using arterial clips and ties. The periosteum is then elevated laterally from the anterior surface of the maxilla as far as the infraorbital foramen but no further. Superiorly this sub periosteal dissection is continued into the orbit. The dissection will expose the anterior lacrimal crest and lacrimal sack and also the anterior ethmoid artery. The lacrimal sac is dissected free of the lacrimal fossa and the duct lifted upward to allow its division which is done as distally as is possible to aid lacrimal drainage after surgery. The periosteum is carefully elevated around the anterior ethmoid artery until sufficient length is exposed to allow it to be either clipped with liga clips or diathermied using bipolar diathermy before being divided. This is an extremely important landmark as it is at the level of the cribriform plate. The orbital dissection is then continued back to the posterior ethmoid artery which lies close to the optic foramen. Dissection does not normally proceed posterior to this point and it is not usually necessary to divide the posterior ethmoid artery in order to perform the procedure.

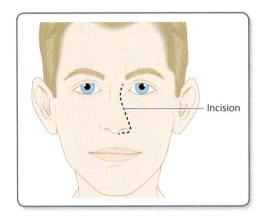

Figure 10.3 Incision for lateral rhinotomy approach.

Inferiorly the incision is carried through the nasal groove exposing the piriform aperture and nasal cavity. The freed alar cartilage can be retracted using a traction suture providing maximal exposure of the nasal cavity.

An antrostomy can be made if necessary to inspect the extent of the tumor in the maxilla and orbital floor. It is made in the anterior wall of the maxilla using a burr or if preferred a hammer, gouge and bone nibblers.

The first osteotomy connects the antrostomy with the nasal cavity and is made horizontally at the level of the floor of the maxillary antrum (**Figure 10.2**). If an antrostomy has not been made the osteotomy is made laterally through the anterior wall of the maxilla to a point just medial to the vertical level of the infraorbital foramen. This is best performed with an oscillating saw or a sharp osteotome. The osteotomy is continued posteriorly at the level of the floor of the nasal cavity back along the lateral nasal wall until the pterygoid plates are reached. This is best accomplished with a sharp osteotome but can be performed using bone nibbling forceps. If using a hammer and osteotome the sound becomes more solid as the pterygoid plates are reached.

The second osteotomy is made vertically from the antrostomy (or the lateral extent of the horizontal osteotomy if an antrostomy has not been made) up to and through the inferior orbital rim medial to the infraorbital foramen. This is made using an oscillating saw or sharp osteotome. It is continued posteriorly through the orbital floor while the orbital contents are carefully retracted using a malleable copper retractor.

The third osteotomy is again carried out using an oscillating saw and transects the orbital process of the maxilla extending up toward but stopping below the anterior ethmoid foramen. This osteotomy is continued posteriorly in a horizontal plane below the level of the anterior and posterior ethmoid foramen and therefore below the cribriform plate. This antrostomy enters into the ethmoid air cells system and may be performed with either very gentle use of a sharp osteotome or with very small bone nibblers. The osteotomy stops just short of the posterior ethmoid foramen and artery.

The final osteotomy joins this osteotomy running vertically from just in front of the posterior ethmoid foramen down to join the osteotomy which has been previously carried out running back and medially along the orbital floor. This is best accomplished with heavy angled scissors and separates the specimen from the pterygoid plates. This is the point at which bleeding is most likely but by sequencing the osteotomies in this manner the specimen can be removed and the bleeding controlled initially by packing and then by use of electrocautery. If there is significant bleeding from bone edges then bone wax can be used to control this.

If there are concerns about surgical margins at this point specimens can be sent for frozen section to enable the best possible clearance of tumor.

It is not usually necessary to pack the cavity after surgery but if there are concerns about bleeding then a pack of ribbon gauze soaked in Whitehead's varnish can be applied and removed the following day. The skin edges are carefully approximated using fine sutures to achieve the least conspicuous scar. The tarsorrhaphy suture is removed.

Postoperatively the patient's visual acuity is checked. Temporary diplopia is quite common and usually settles with conservative management.

Patients are told that they would expect some initially increased mucus discharge with some blood. They are also told that they are likely to experience significant crusting particularly in the early weeks after surgery and they are taught how to douche the nose with lukewarm saline solution to help soften and remove the crusts. Nursing staff are told to be watchful for significant bleeding and also the signs of meningitis.

Further reading

McGuirt WF. Maxillectomy. Otolaryngol Clin North Am 1995; 28:1175–89.

Myers EN. Medial maxillectomy. In: Myers EN (ed.), Operative Otolaryngology: Head and Neck Surgery, 2nd edn. Philadelphia, PA: Saunders Elsevier, 2008.

Shah JP, Patel S, Singh B (eds.) Jatin Shah's Head and Neck Surgery and Oncology, 4th edn. Philadelphia, PA: Mosby Elsevier, 2012.

Wassef SF, Batra PS, Barnett S. Skull base inverted papilloma: a comprehensive review. ISRN Surg 2012; 2012:175–903.

Maxillectomy

Nicholas Stafford

Introduction

A total maxillectomy is one of a minority of head and neck procedures that can have a profound effect on the patient's appearance and function.

First performed successfully by Syme in 1828, total maxillectomy forms the cornerstone of a number of surgical operations described for tumors of the nasal cavity and paranasal sinuses. This chapter describes the classic operation and orbital exenteration.

Preoperative considerations

Most nasal/sinonasal malignancies are at an advanced stage at presentation. Some will already be incurable. Following a careful clinical assessment and biopsy of the lesion accurate imaging, preferably with both CT and MRI, will facilitate effective treatment planning.

If orbital involvement necessitates an orbital exenteration then this must be discussed with the patient. Often such extensive disease is indicative of widespread extension into other, adjacent tissues and consequently, unlikely curability.

All patients require preoperative referral to a prosthetic orthodontist so that a dental impression of the upper jaw can be taken and a dental plate fashioned. This will be the first step in the provision of a permanent plate and obturator. Again, the patient should be made fully aware of this long-term necessity.

A neck dissection is not indicated unless there is substantive clinical and/or radiological evidence of disease.

Staging

T staging for carcinomas of the maxillary sinus is:
- T1 tumor linked to mucosa of the maxillary sinus with no erosion or destruction of bone
- T2 tumor with bone erosion or destruction extending into the hard palate and/or middle nasal meatus, except extension into the posterior maxillary sinus wall or pterygoid plates
- T3 tumor invades any of the following: posterior wall of sinus, subcutaneous tissues, floor of medial wall of orbit, pterygoid fossa, ethmoid sinus
- T4a tumor invades anterior orbit, skin of cheek, pterygoid plates, infra-temporal fossa, cribriform plate, sphenoid, or frontal sinus
- T4b tumor invades orbital apex, dura, brain, cranial nerve (other than V2) nasopharynx, or clivus

Antibiotics

These should be started preoperatively and continued for 5 days postoperatively.

Anesthetic considerations

The patient is intubated using an ET tube introduced through the contralateral nasal airway. A nasogastric feeding tube (NGT) should also be introduced. Unless the operation is complicated by excessive hemorrhage, a tracheostomy is not required.

Operative technique

- A Weber-Ferguson incision is employed (**Figure 11.1**). The lateral, horizontal element runs approximately 3 mm below the margin of the lower lid: too close and an ectropion is likely: further away and lower lid edema is a problem. Try and make the angle between this and the vertical portion of the incision at the medial canthus as obtuse as possible to avoid skin tip necrosis
- The upper lip is divided in the midline
- From the point where the lip incision extends intraorally to the frenulum of upper lip, this incision is then extended horizontally and laterally in the gingivo buccal sulcus to a point just behind the maxillary tuberosity (**Figure 11.2**)
- Leaving the orbicularis muscle intact, the periosteum of the inferior orbital rim is incised down to bone, facilitating the raising of the flap laterally
- The infraorbital nerve and vessels will need to be divided where they exit the infraorbital foramen
- The cheek skin flap is then raised off the anterior face of the maxilla as far lateral at the medial end of the zygomatic arch

- From the upper lip frenulum a second, midline, mucosal incision is made posteriorly to the junction of the hard and soft palate
- This incision is then taken laterally, along the posterior margin of the hard palate, to join the other mucosal incision immediately

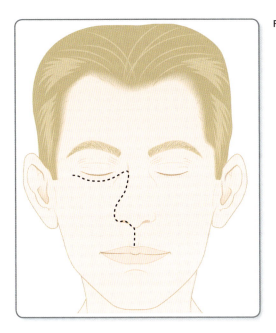

Figure 11.1 A Weber-Ferguson incision.

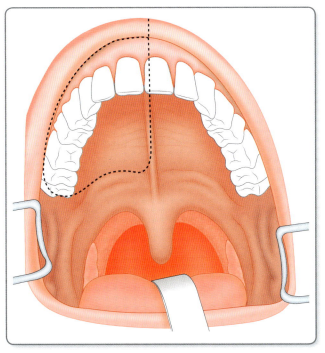

Figure 11.2 Weber-Ferguson incision extending intraorally to the frenulum of the upper lip, then extended horizontally and laterally in the gingivo buccal sulcus to a point just behind the maxillary tuberosity.

behind the maxillary tuberosity. Unless oncologically essential, the soft palate should not be split

- The orbital periosteum is raised off the bony floor of the orbit so as to expose the anterior part of the inferior orbital fissure
- The lateral bony attachments of the maxilla are divided using an oscillating saw. The temporal process of the zygomatic bone is divided vertically: the frontal process is divided horizontally, just above the level of the zygomatic arch, the cut extending through to the lateral margin of the infraorbital fissure (**Figure 11.3**)
- While gently retracting the globe superiorly a further osteotomy is created from the infraorbital fissure medially to the apex of the pyriform aperture of the nose (**Figure 11.3**)
- Following removal of the ipsilateral first upper incisor, the hard palate is then divided anteroposteriorly. This is best undertaken with an oscillating saw. If possible, this osteotomy lies just lateral to the midline so that the nasal septum can be preserved intact, assuming it is not involved by tumor
- The medial wall of the maxilla/lateral wall of the nasal cavity is divided horizontally just above the level of the middle turbinate
- Use a curved osteotome behind the tuberosity of the maxilla to separate the maxilla from the pterygoid plates; the maxilla can now be fully mobilized
- Using curved Mayo or McIndoe scissors to divide residual soft tissue attachments the maxillary block can now be removed

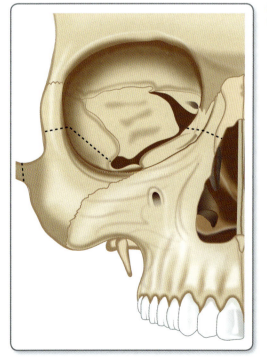

Figure 11.3 Osteotomies for a standard right maxillectomy.

- Following temporary packing of the cavity, hemostasis can now be achieved, the maxillary artery being tied or clipped where it lies in the soft tissues posteriorly
- Once dry, the cavity and inner aspect of the cheek skin flap should be lined with a quilted split thickness skin graft. This will speed up its epithlialization and help prevent cheek contracture and the possibility of an ugly upper lip 'snarl' deformity
- The cavity is then packed with gauze impregnated with Bismuth iodine paraffin paste or Whitehead's varnish and the temporary dental plate wired in using circumzygomatic wires
- The wound is closed in layers, paying particular attention to accurate reconstruction of the vermillion border of the lip

Postoperative care

The temporary antral pack should be removed under a general anesthetic and the cavity cleaned 7–10 days later. Once the cavity is infection free and has re-epithelialized, a permanent dental plate and obturator can be fitted.

Oral feeding can usually commence on the second or third postoperative day, the NGT being removed at that time.

In the unirradiated patient, skin sutures can be removed after 1 week: postradiotherapy, allow 2 weeks. The angled junction at the medial canthus is a common site of minor wound breakdown after this procedure.

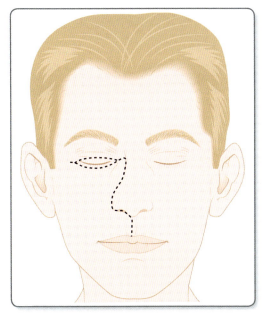

Figure 11.4 A Weber-Ferguson incision with an additional upper lid incision removing the tarsal plate.

Orbital extenteration

- A Weber-Ferguson incision is employed, with an additional upper lid incision removing the tarsal plate (**Figure 11.4**)
- An incision is made through the periosteum along the edge of the supraorbital rim
- Elevating this periosteum anteroposteriorly, the orbit can now be mobilized, from above down. Stay in the subperiosteal plane
- The medial and lateral suspensory ligaments are divided
- At the orbital apex a Lahey clip or equivalent is used to clamp the optic nerve and ophthalmic artery which are then divided
- An osteotomy is made posteriorly across the bony floor of the orbit in order to mobilize the maxilla
- The upper and lower lids are stitched together as part of the overall closure

Medial wall maxillectomy

The surgical approach to the lateral wall of the nose/medial wall of the maxilla is via a lateral rhinotomy (see Chapter 10). This procedure was first described by Michaux in 1848 but popularized by Moure in 1902.

Medial wall maxillectomy is an effective surgical procedure for tumors localized to the lateral wall of the nose and also provides excellent access for certain nasopharyngeal tumors, e.g. juvenile angiofibroma. It can also be modified to allow good access to tumors of the nasal septum.

Further reading

De Souza C, Gil Z, Fliss DM. Atlas of Head and Neck Surgery. New Delhi: Jaypee Brothers Medical, Publishers (P) Ltd, 2013.

Anterior skull base (including pituitary fossa) tumors

Ashis Pathak and Bruce Mathew

Common tumors of the anterior skull base

Anterior skull base tumors can be divided into two groups depending on tumors arising from the bones of the cranium; and the anterior cranial floor, sellar and parasellar region, infratemporal fossa, paranasal sinuses, and orbit.

Classification of lesions of the anterior skull base

Skull base meningiomas
- En plaque with underlying hyperostosis
- Olfactory groove
- Planum sphenoidale
- Tuberculum sella
- Sphenoid wing: lateral, middle, and medial (sphenocavernous)
- Infiltrating : involving cavernous sinus, paranasal sinus and/or infratemporal fossa

Cartilaginous and bony lesions
- Chondroma
- Chondrosarcoma
- Chordoma
- Fibrous dysplasia
- Osteogenic sarcoma

Sellar/parasellar/nasopharyngeal/paranasal lesions
- Pituitary tumor
- Craniopharyngioma

- Angiofibroma
- Carcinomas involving skull base

Miscellaneous

- Esthesioneuroblastoma
- Lymphoma
- Metastasis

Evaluation of the patient

Detailed history

- Duration, progress of symptoms, extent of disability
- Neurological evaluation: Extent of deficit – partial or complete
- Progress of symptoms and signs
- Image findings on computerized tomography (CT), computerized axial angiography (CTA), magnetic resonance imaging (MRI), magnetic resonance angiography (MRA), digital subtraction angiography (DSA)
- Comorbidities
- Fitness to undergo general anesthesia
- Risks involved in surgical resection

Intraoperative monitoring

- Hemodynamic status
- Cranial nerve function monitoring
- EEG
- In infiltrating tumors
  - Barbiturate coma
  - Hypothermia
  - Somatosensory-evoked potentials
  - Brain stem-evoked potentials

Planning of surgery

Clear anatomical concept – based on:
- Location of lesion
- Neurovascular involvement
- Extent of distortion of normal anatomical structures

Subspecialty team work planning

- Need for a single approach/combined approach or staged approach
- Preoperative embolization of the lesion may be done as per surgeon's choice
- Vascular bypass surgery for lesions needing radical resection involving great vessels
- Image guidance radiology

Reconstruction plan

- Dural based repair
- Fat plug for small holes

- Reinforcement with vascularized tissue/flap
- Myocutaneous flap for larger defect
- Harvested bone graft for reconstruction
- Prosthetic implant for reconstructing the defect

Postoperative care

- To be nursed in intensive care or high dependency unit under care of neurointensivist
- Monitoring of hemodynamic and electrolyte status
- Assessment of related cranial nerves to look for impairment
- Post op CT scan to look for symptomatic or asymptomatic hematoma, brain swelling or pneumocephalus
- Postoperative transcranial doppler (TCD)/DSA to look for patency of vascular graft
- Detection of cerebrospinal fluid (CSF) leak or wound related problems, especially in the case of repeat surgery or irradiated patients

Frontobasal approach

This approach was described by Sekhar et al (1992) (**Figure 12.1**).

Indications

Tumors/lesions in
- Anterior skull base
- Sellar/suprasellar region
- Dorsum sella
- Clivus

Advantages

- Reconstruction possible
- Pericranial/galeal-frontalis muscle/microvascular free flap

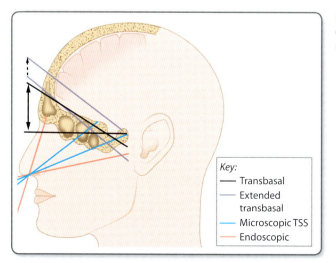

Figure 12.1 Trajectory and extent of anatomical exposure for various skull base approaches.

Key:
— Transbasal
— Extended transbasal
— Microscopic TSS
— Endoscopic

- Can be done in conjunction with a transfacial approach for lesions involving infracranial compartments

Limitations

- Limited by optic nerves and carotid arteries posteriorly
- Olfactory function may be compromised by large skull base lesions
- Needs effective reconstruction for lesions invading skull base

Technique

- In large lesions with associated brain swelling a lumbar drain may be inserted for possible CSF drainage to reduce intracranial pressure (ICP)
- Under general anesthesia (GA) the patient is placed in a supine position with head elevation of 30°
- A bicoronal incision is planned from the preauricular area extending from one zygomatic arch to the other running behind the coronal suture (**Figure 12.2**)
- Scalp flap dissected up to the supraorbital rim and frontonasal suture
- Supraorbital nerves must be preserved, as they may lie in a notch or bony canal
- A bifrontal craniotomy is performed
- Using a reciprocating saw the anterior portion of the orbital roof along with bilateral supraorbital rim can be removed

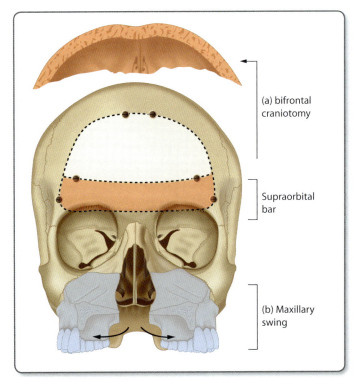

Figure 12.2 (a) Bifrontal craniotomy (red) and (b) maxillary swing procedure (blue).

(a) bifrontal craniotomy

Supraorbital bar

(b) Maxillary swing

- Under direct vision the midline dura is incised bilaterally, and the anterior end of the superior sagittal sinus lodged in the anterior falx coagulated and resected after ligation
- If dura is very tense the lumbar drain is opened and CSF drained to reduce the ICP
- A bilateral dural flap is raised by incising the dura mater horizontally parallel to the base
- The crista galli is excised
- The dural sleeve around the olfactory groove is incised
- The anterior and posterior ethmoidal arteries are coagulated
- Lesions located in the anterior skull base can now be visualized and excised piecemeal using coagulation diathermy or a Cavitron ultrasonic aspirator
- Depending on the location of the lesion the frontal lobes are retracted with intact dura (for extradural lesions) or after a durotomy (for intradural lesions)
- Using a high-speed air drill the following areas can be drilled:
  - Bone over the carotid canal to decompress the optic nerves
  - Bone over the middle and posterior ethmoid sinuses to gain access into the ethmoid and sphenoid air cells
- After excision of the lesion the anterior cranial base is reconstructed and the dura is repaired

Combined approaches

These approaches are meant for lesions extending/encroaching into different anatomical confines in and around the skull base, especially tumors invading inferiorly. The exposures have to be made to gain access to different compartments to allow for en bloc resection.

Fronto-orbito zygomatic osteotomy approach

This approach was described by Sindou and Alawan (1990).

Indications

- For lesions involving anterior skull base, sphenoid, parasellar region and involving infratemporal fossa

Advantages

Apart from better exposure it has the advantage of:
- Minimal retraction of brain
- Being able to combine with other approaches for lesions extending inferiorly and posteriorly
- Scope for using vascularized temporalis muscle flap in reconstruction

Limitations

- Lesion invading through the medial skull base

Technique

- A coronal or curvilinear incision is made starting below the zygomatic arch and 2 mm in front of tragus in order to preserve

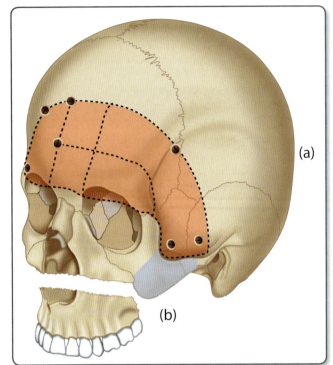

Figure 12.3 (a) Fronto-orbital zygomatic approach (zygomatic arch removed [blue area]) and (b) Le Fort 1 osteotomy.

(a)

(b)

branches of facial nerve and the superficial temporal artery (**Figure 12.3**)

- The scalp flap is raised taking care to preserve the facial nerve branches by staying below the periosteal plane between the superficial and deep layer of the temporalis fascia. The dissection is carried forward and downward to expose the zygomatic bone, the frontal bone up to the supraorbital rim and the temporal bone covered by the temporalis muscle and fascia
- A fronto temporal craniotomy is performed
- The dura is lifted off the orbital roof, pterion and middle fossa floor and the periorbita is separated from the adjacent orbital roof
- Using a reciprocating saw the medial part of supraorbital rim is incised protecting the periorbita and the dura mater with appropriately sized retractors. The orbital roof and lateral wall of orbit is excised up to 2.5–3 cm posteriorly
- The zygomatic bone is incised horizontally through the frontozygomatic process, the zygomatic suture is incised and the zygomatic arch is incised posteriorly close to the condylar fossa
- Reconstruction is carried out after dural closure using the original durotomy leaves or dural substitute, e.g. pericranial or temporalis fascia graft or artificial dura
- Open sinuses may be packed with fat graft and tissue glue

- If available a long vascularized pericranial flap or temporalis muscle flap may be helpful for reconstruction. For very large cavities vascularized rectus abdominis flap may be used
- In case of a big bony defect a split thickness pericranial bone graft or a contoured prosthetic device can be used for reconstruction, particularly for intraosseous orbitosphenoidal meningiomas

Craniofacial approach

This approach was described by Cocke et al (1990).

Indications

- Anterior skull base tumors extending to ethmoid sinus, infraorbital region, and infratemporal fossa laterally

Advantages

- Helps adequate resection of tumors extending to midface region
- Access to the lesion is direct with no major structures in the way
- Can be combined with cranial approach for extensive and invasive lesions

Disadvantages

- Cosmetic risks even though healing is good normally

Technique

- The patient is intubated using an oral tube
- A lateral rhinotomy incision is used on the side of the tumor as shown (**Figure 12.4**)
- The incision can be extended
  - Inferiorly, up to the nasal sill in the midline and then splitting the upper lip
  - Superiorly, in the lateral direction going subciliary or transconjunctival
- A maxillotomy is made taking care to preserve the infraorbital nerve unless it is involved by the lesion
- Using a reciprocating saw a medial maxillotomy is performed by making a horizontal cut in the maxilla to the lateral wall of nose and vertical cut through the orbital floor medially and horizontally
- The palate is to be split in the midline allowing the maxilla to be swung laterally (Figure 12.2)
- The lesion is debulked/excised taking care to control any bleeding from the sphenopalatine artery
- Combined with cranial exposure a dural defect may need to be repaired using vascularized pericranial flap raised with the cranial incision
- Repositioning of the maxilla is carried out using miniplates and screws
- A lumbar drain may be needed for controlling ICP and managing CSF leaks

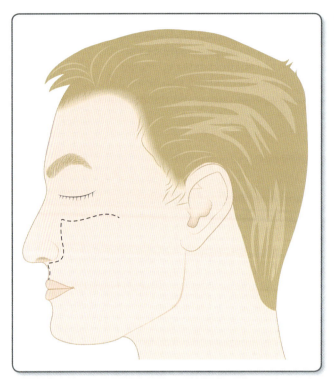

Figure 12.4 Incision for transfacial approaches.

- Postoperatively a palate splint may be needed for 4–6 weeks to support the reconstruction till it heals

Midface degloving approach

This approach was described by Price (1986).

Indications

- For tumors involving anterior skull base, clivus, and nasopharynx

Advantages

- Wider bilateral exposure
- Avoidance of facial scar

Disadvantages

- Postoperative synechiae and stenosis of the nasal aperture

Technique

- The mucosa of the nose is incised circumferentially anterior to the cartilaginous septum
- Lifting the upper lip an incision is made around the upper gingivio-labial mucosa with the lateral extension of the incision over the anterolateral face of each maxillary sinus
- The anterior nasal bone is exposed as the soft tissue is lifted
- This allows further exposure in the form of:

- Bilateral medial maxillotomies to have a wide exposure for removal of extensive midline craniofacial lesions (**Figure 12.2**)
- LeForte I type exposure that is made by incising the upper jaw horizontally above the level of the roots of the teeth and their nerve distribution (**Figure 12.3**)
- After tumor removal reconstruction is achieved using mini titanium plates and screws taking care to maintain the natural alignment of the teeth
- The mucosa is sutured back and a nasal pack or splint may be needed to support healing of palate

Approach to the sella and upper clivus

Transnasal approach (Figure 12.1)

Indications

- For lesions involving sella-supra-sellar region, sphenoid sinus, midline clivus

Advantages

- Minimal distortion of anatomy
- Cosmetically most acceptable
- No handling of brain
- Hospital stay and recovery quicker

Disadvantages

- Limited exposure
- Cannot approach laterally invasive lesions
- CSF leak common
- Difficult to repair dural breach

Technique

- The patient is orally intubated
- Combination of cocaine and nasal decongestant applied to nasal cavity for 20 minutes before start of anesthesia
- The patient put supine with the head facing the surgeon
- Alternatively the head may be extended and the surgeon may prefer to stand at the head end of the patient
- The C-arm of the image intensifier is stationed so as to have a lateral view of the sella turcica avoiding parallax error
- This guides the surgeon to the sella and adjoining region during surgery
- Under X-ray guidance the anterior wall of sella is identified and after coagulating the overlying mucosa it is incised near the midline septal area
- Using a speculum the bony septum is fractured to the opposite side and the keel of the vomer with the adjoining bone exposed
    Alternatively:
    - The nasal mucosa is incised over the cartilaginous septum and the nasal cartilage is dissected free on one side

- - As dissection proceeds the nasal speculum is advanced dissecting the septal mucosa on both the side of bony nasal septum (as per and old fashioned submucosal resection of the septum)
  - The bony septum is excised
- Using a bone forceps, the keel of the vomer including the anterior wall of sphenoid sinus is excised
- The opening in the sphenoid sinus is enlarged to allow instrumentation of intrasinus lesions
- The bony floor of the sella is fractured/drilled and using fine up cut punches the opening of the bony sellar floor is enlarged
- In case of lesions extending into the clival region, the clival area is verified by X-ray and drilled using a high-speed drill
- The sellar floor/clival dura comes into view
- The dura is coagulated and a stellate shaped incision made to expose the lesion
- After excision of the lesion hemostasis is ensured using floseal and fibrillar sponge
- In case of major CSF leak use of harvested fat/fascia along with glue is helpful
- The nasal cavity is packed with expandable nasal tampons
- However if bleeding is minimal the nasal cavity can be left unpacked

Endoscopic endonasal approach to anterior skull base and sella (Figure 12.1)

Minimally invasive surgery is an emerging trend that holds a great promise for the future, whereby vast majority of lesions would be excised under direct endoscopy or as an endoscopy-assisted procedure (Prosser et al. 2012, Zador & Gnanalingham 2013).

Indications

For lesions involving or extending to the:
- Sphenoethmoidal sinus
- Sellar and or suprasellar regions
- Planum sphenoidale and/or cribiform plate
- Frontal sinus
- Pterygoid region
- Infratemporal region

Advantages

- Improved visualization of structures
- Minimal distortion of normal anatomy
- Increasing efficiency in viewing hidden anatomy
- Can be combined with cranial resection
- Cosmetically better

Disadvantages

- Steep learning curve
- Narrow corridor of access
- Higher chance of CSF leak in lesions involving the dura mater

Preoperative planning

High-resolution CT provides good outline of bony, vascular and soft tissue anatomy.

Fusion of MRI with CT scan pictures gives good orientation. The patient must be free from any nasal infection.

Optical tracking system with registration based on fiducial is helpful.

Technique

- Under GA the head is fixed in a three-pin fixation system
- The neck is extended and the extension is dependent on the location of the lesion, the maximum extension being for lesions in the anterior skull base and frontal sinus region
- Nasal decongestion is achieved by topical use of cocaine or oxymetazoline
- Two surgeon, four-hand technique is useful for creating an optimal corridor and removal of skull base lesions
- In lesions needing repair of a large dural defect a large nasoseptal mucoperiosteal flap is harvested and temporarily tucked in the nasopharynx for subsequent use
- The nasal corridor is created as required, by excision of:
  - One or both middle turbinates
  - Bony nasal septum
  - Sphenoidectomy/ethmoidectomy
  - Bony skull base adjacent to the lesion
- For sellar lesions the bony floor of the sella is adequately drilled and the exposed dural lining is coagulated and incised. This is followed by tumor excision under endoscopic guidance
- For an anterior skull base lesion any feeding vessel is coagulated before or after the dura is exposed
- Tumor removal is done by initial debulking followed by coagulation and mobilization of the tumor capsule
- Any adherent important structure is separated or coagulated under direct endoscopic visualization
- Reconstruction of the defect in the anterior skull base floor is undertaken using an in-lay of artificial dural patch followed by the on-lay of a vascularized mucoperiosteal flap harvested earlier. This is supported by the inflated bulb of a Foley's catheter for 5 days approximately

Management of a CSF leak

In cases of persistent CSF leak that does not show signs of abatement the following strategy should be followed:

- An initial CT scan of head to look for established pneumocephalus
- If there is no pneumocephalus, insert lumbar drain and have controlled CSF drainage depending on the tolerance of the patient for 3 days. Also watch for fluid and electrolyte imbalance. Once CSF leak stops for 48 hours clamp the lumbar drain to give a challenge which, if successful, is followed by removal of the drain

- In case of gross pneumocephalus or no improvement of the CSF leak with a lumbar drain an open repair of the leakage site has to be carried out using a vascularized flap

Antibiotic policy

The antibiotic regime should be given as follows:
1. For all trans-sphenoidal and endonasal endoscopic cases without major breach or CSF leak only perioperative antibiotic cover is indicated
2. For extensive combined intra and extracranial procedures involving air spaces or nasal cavity:
   a. Perioperative antibiotic to be to be repeated 4 hourly over the first 24 hours
   b. Postoperative antibiotic for 3 days or until the CSF drain is removed
3. For re-explorations, three postoperative days of antibiotic therapy should be enough
4. For uncontrolled CSF leaks no antibiotic prophylaxis is recommended but close monitoring is needed to detect evidence of meningitis that would require appropriate treatment.

Further reading

Sekhar LN, Sen CN, Snyderman CN, Janecka IP. Anterior, anterolateral and lateral approaches to extradural clival tumours. In: Sekhar LN, Janecka IP (eds), Surgery of Cranial Base Tumours. New York: Raven Press, 1992.

References

Cocke EW, Robertson JH, Robertson JT, Cook JP. The extended maxillotomy and subtotal maxillotomy for excision of skull base tumours. Arch Otolaryngol Head Neck Surg 1990; 116:92–104.

Price JC. The midfacial degloving approach to central skull base. Ear Nose Throat J 1986; 65:174–80.

Prosser JD, Vender JR, Alleyne CH, Solares CA. Expanded endoscopic endonasal approaches to skull base meningiomas. J Neurol Surg B Skull Base 2012; 73:147–56.

Sekhar LN, Nanda A, Sen CN, Snyderman CN, Janecka IP. The extended frontal approach to tumors of the anterior, middle, and posterior skull base. J Neurosurgery 1992; 76:198–206.

Sindou M, Alawan M. Orbital and/or zygomatic removal in an approach to lesions near the cranial base. Surgical technic, anatomic study and analysis of a series of 24 cases. Neurochirurgie 1990; 36:225–33.

Zador Z, Gnanalingham K. Endoscopic transnasal approach to the pituitary – operative technique and nuances. Br J Neurosurg 2013;27: 718-26.

13 Application of endoscopic sinus surgery in head and neck oncology

Robin Youngs, Tang Ing Ping and Narayanan Prepageran

The development and refinement of endoscopic approaches to the paranasal sinuses in the management of chronic rhinosinusitis has allowed these same techniques to be used in the assessment and treatment of neoplastic conditions of the nasal cavity, paranasal sinuses and anterior skull base.

There are a number of advantages that endoscopic approaches have over traditional external approaches:

- Purely endoscopic access avoids disfiguring facial incisions (Batra et al. 2005). When an external approach is required the use of an adjunctive endoscopic approach can decrease the size of the external incision required
- Overall morbidity of surgery and length of hospital stay is reduced
- Control of vascular supply to neoplasms can be obtained closer to the pathology with ready access to the maxillary, sphenoplatine, and ethmoid vessels

The principle of en bloc resection of paranasal sinus neoplasms has been challenged with the advent of endoscopic approaches (Luong et al. 2010). By its nature endoscopic excision has to be largely piecemeal. The character of paranasal sinus neoplasia, however, is conducive to a piecemeal approach. Of prime importance is the determination of the origin of the neoplasm (Lawson & Patel 2009). Many paranasal sinus neoplasms have a relatively narrow base. Assessment with endoscopy and radiology can be used to determine the origin and extent of tumor and hence tailor an endoscopic approach to maximize the potential for control and minimize complications and morbidity.

From an anatomical perspective the extent of endoscopic dissection required depends on the location, extent and histological characteristics of the neoplasm. In this way a number of discreet approaches can be described:

1. Nasal cavity – a limited approach for small benign lesions confined to the nasal cavity
2. Endoscopic medial maxillectomy – for lesions originating from the maxillary sinus
3. Endoscopic frontoethmoidal approaches – for anterior lesions
4. Endoscopic posterior approaches – for lesions in the posterior ethmoid and sphenoid sinuses
5. Endoscopic lateral approaches – when lesions adjacent to the paranasal sinuses are accessed through the sinuses. Examples would be pathology in the pterygopalatine fossa and removal of pituitary tumors

Preoperative considerations

Accurate imaging is vital in planning the appropriate approach. Computerized tomographic (CT) images are essential to assess anatomical variation, extent of disease and bony erosion (**Figure 13.1**). In oncological sinus surgery MR images are also important in determining soft tissue involvement and distinguishing between tumor and secondary mucosal disease (Maroldi et al. 1997). The use of image-guided surgery (IGS) using navigational systems is also standard in many centers, although their use is limited by financial considerations (Doshi & Youngs 2007). The most modern IGS technology allows for intraoperative CT scanning in order to update the operative image. Fusion of CT and MR images by IGS systems is also possible. For vascular lesions angiography including magnetic resonance angiography (MRA) can be required, including the use of preoperative tumor embolization to reduce intra-operative blood loss.

A preoperative tumor biopsy to obtain histological confirmation of diagnosis is necessary. The ultimate diagnosis must be made taking clinical and radiological findings into consideration as a biopsy taken from the nasal cavity may not be entirely representative of deeper tumor in the paranasal sinuses. In highly vascular lesions such as the angiofibroma biopsy can result in major hemorrhage. In such cases diagnosis can be made based on clinical and radiological findings and confirmed following resection. Intraoperative analysis by frozen-section is also required in many cases to assess completeness of resection.

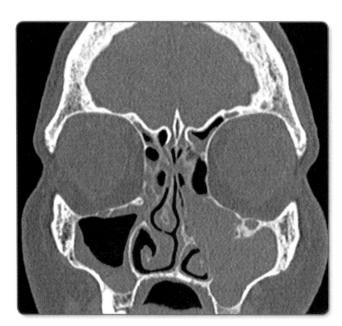

Figure 13.1 Coronal CT scan showing opacity of the left maxillary antrum in a case of inverted papilloma.

Consent for surgery

There are a number of potential complications which the patient must be made aware of. The likelihood of complications will depend on the location and extent of surgery. In experienced hands the incidence of major complications should be minimal. When undertaking more extensive resections for malignant disease some postoperative deficit can be inevitable and must be discussed fully with the patient:

- Intraoperative and postoperative bleeding, which may require nasal packing
- Injury to skull base and CSF leak
- Injury to orbital structures, including visual loss due to optic nerve damage and diplopia caused by injury to extraocular muscles, particularly the medial rectus. Diplopia can also occur with removal of the bony support of the (medial) orbital wall
- Epiphora due to trauma to the nasolacrimal duct
- Postoperative loss of sense of smell
- Postoperative crusting
- Dental and facial anesthesia due to damage to the infraorbital nerve and its branches

Anesthetic considerations

Anesthetic planning will depend on preoperative comorbidities. In addition, projected length of procedure and estimated blood loss will be taken into account. Endoscopic surgery will be facilitated by controlled hypotension. In addition, the use of local anesthetic infiltration and topical vasoconstriction can improve the surgical conditions.

Endoscopic medial maxillectomy

This procedure facilitates access to the maxillary sinus (**Figure 13.2**). From a technical perspective, the anterior wall and inferior part of the sinus are less accessible. It should be noted that the most inferior part of the sinus is below the level of the nasal floor. The procedure involves removal of the inferior turbinate, part of the frontal process of the maxilla and the parts of the ethmoid complex that comprise the medial antral wall. The most frequent pathology treated by this approach is the inverted papilloma.

Operative technique

- The nasal cavity is inspected endoscopically to assess anatomy and pathology

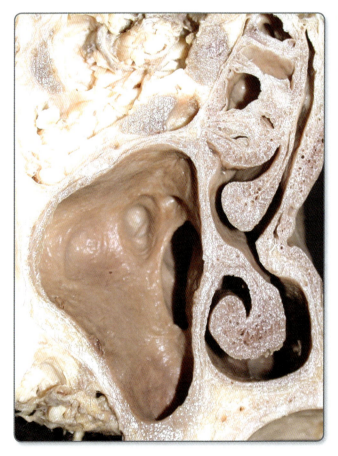

Figure 13.2 Coronal cadaver section demonstrating the right maxillary sinus and its relationships to the nasal cavity and ethmoidal sinuses.

- If the nasal cavity contains tumor to the extent of obscuring anatomical structures the tumor can be debulked. This can be facilitated with the use of a powered microdebrider
- An uncinectomy is performed and the natural ostium of the maxillary sinus identified
- The maxillary ostium is widened posteriorly by removing the posterior fontanelle to a point level with the posterior wall of the sinus in the A–P plane. With this maneuver bleeding from the sphenopalatine artery may have to be controlled with bipolar diathermy
- The frontal process of the maxilla can be identified by its surface marking, the maxillary line. This bone can be removed by punch forceps or a diamond burr, exposing the underlying lacrimal sac. Incision and marsupialization of the lacrimal sac may reduce the incidence of postoperative epiphora
- The inferior turbinate is removed longitudinally. The mucosa of the inferior meatus can be elevated inferiorly toward the floor of the nasal cavity exposing the underlying bone. This bone is removed with a diamond burr until it is level with the nasal floor
- The maxillary sinus can be visualized with 30°, 45°, and 70° angled endoscopes. Tumor and diseased mucosa can be removed. Underlying bone can be drilled with a diamond burr
- For lesions arising from the anterior sinus wall access can be improved by an anterior septotomy, allowing approach from the contralateral nostril. This can be undertaken using either a septal window or a hemitransfixion incision. In this way the angle of access to the maxillary sinus can be improved (Ramakrishnan et al. 2011)
- At the end of the procedure hemostasis is obtained. Many surgeons are now using absorbable nasal packing to avoid the postoperative discomfort of packing requiring later removal

Endoscopic frontoethmoidal approaches

Standard endoscopic approaches to the ethmoidal and frontal sinuses can be used in the treatment of neoplastic lesions (**Figure 13.3**). Neoplasms conducive to this approach will almost always be benign, with inverted papilloma, hemangiomas and osteomas being the most common examples. The creation of a large surgical cavity following tumor removal facilitates endoscopic follow-up (**Figure 13.4**). For lesions involving the frontal sinus extended approaches such as the modified Lothrop or Draf type III procedures can provide wide access.

Operative technique (modified Lothrop procedure)

- The nasal cavity is inspected endoscopically to assess anatomy and pathology
- If the nasal cavity contains tumor to the extent of obscuring anatomical structures the tumor can be debulked. This can be facilitated with the use of a powered microdebrider

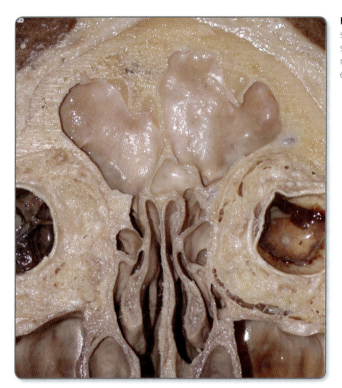

Figure 13.3 Coronal cadaver section showing the frontal sinus and its relationships to the nasal septum, orbit and anterior ethmoidal sinuses.

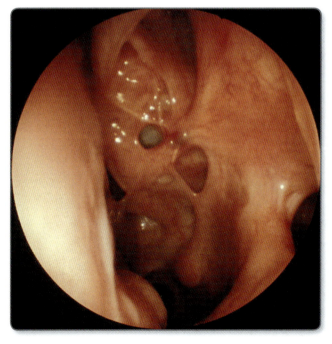

Figure 13.4 Endoscopic view into surgically created left ethmoidal cavity 6 months following excision of an anterior ethmoidal inverted papilloma.

- The part of the perpendicular plate of the ethmoid bone that forms the bony part of the anterior-superior nasal septum below the floor of the frontal sinus is removed with mucosal preservation
- Access to the frontal sinus itself can be facilitated by the use of 'mini-trephination.' This technique allows irrigation of the frontal sinus from above
- The posterior wall of the frontal sinus must be identified, as behind this structure lies the cribriform plate and intracranial contents
- The 'frontonasal beak' bone can be removed anteriorly as far as the skin overlying the nasal bones
- A large median ostium is thereby created facilitating tumor removal and postoperative follow-up
- These procedures are facilitated by the use of angled endoscopes, powered instrumentation and image-guided technology

Endoscopic posterior approach for juvenile angiofibromas

Juvenile nasopharyngeal angiofibroma (JNA) originates from the posterolateral wall of the nasal cavity in close proximity to the superior aspect of the sphenopalatine foramen. These tumors may extend from the nasal cavity to the nasopharynx, paranasal sinuses, the orbit, the pterygopalatine fossa and the infratemporal fossa. Occasionally tumor invasion may occur into the skull base or intracranially (**Figure 13.5**)

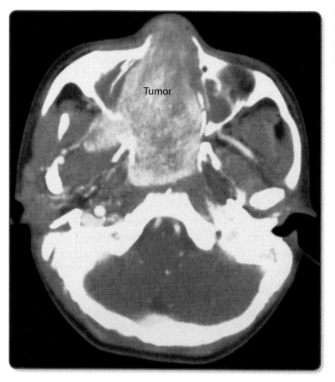

Figure 13.5 Coronal CT scan showing extensive juvenile angiofibroma with skull base and intracranial extension.

Tumor

(Hackman et al. 2009, Zanation et al. 2012). It is important that endoscopic surgeons familiarize themselves with the relative endoscopic anatomical position of the origin and the spread of a JNA as well as the vascular supply of the tumor, with the assistance of preoperative CT scan, MRI, and angiography.

Operative technique

Preoperative angiography and embolization are important to assess the vascularity and feeding vessels of the tumor as well as to reduce bleeding during surgery. Embolization is typically performed 24 hours before scheduled surgery to decrease intraoperative bleeding.

First, the nasal cavity is decongested with Moffat's solution (1 mL of adrenaline 1:1000, 2 mL of 10% cocaine, 4 mL of 8.4% sodium bicarbonate, 13 mL of water/saline) for 20 minutes. Next, the nasal lateral wall especially the attachment of middle turbinate is infiltrated with a solution of lidocaine 0.5-1% with adrenaline 1/100,000 to 1/200,000.

Exposure

The success of the surgery depends on the exposure before manipulation and removal of the angiofibroma.

- A medial maxillectomy is performed to improve the access and to facilitate visualization of the posterior wall of the maxillary sinus and anterior portion of the pterygopalatine fossa (PPF).
- Posterior septectomy is performed to allow for a 'two-nostrils four-hands' surgical technique. Both medial maxillectomy and posterior septectomy are generally assisted by powered instruments
- If there is high risk of exposing bare bone or significant cerebrospinal fluid (CSF) leak at the end of the surgery a nasoseptal rescue flap is raised before the posterior septectomy is performed. A nasoseptal rescue flap consists of elevating the Hadad–Bassagaisteguy nasoseptal flap's (HBF) pedicle but not its paddle (Hadad et al. 2006)
- As these tumors usually fill part of the PPF, a transpterygoid approach to the PPF is always performed with the removal of posterior wall of the maxillary sinus
- After removing the posterior wall of the maxillary sinus, the feeding vessels of the tumor, particularly the sphenopalatine and internal maxillary arteries, are identified, and ligated or cauterized, even after embolization. It should be noted that certain tumors might also have a blood supply from branches of the internal carotid artery and contralateral external carotid artery

Removal of tumor

After these preparatory steps the tumor can now be removed. This depends on the size and extension of the tumor. It is crucial to debulk the intranasal portion of the tumor prior to accessing portions extending beyond sinonasal structures. Tumor debulking is assisted by cutting instruments, bipolar coagulation diathermy, two large bore suction tubes and a powered microdebrider.

- If there is a significant infratemporal fossa extension, an endoscopic Denker's approach is performed to allow access to the junction of lateral and posterior wall of the maxillary sinus. With this approach, the most lateral component of posterior wall of maxillary sinus can be removed
- If the tumor has extended into the orbit, the infraorbital fissure may be accessed via the PPF to remove the orbital portion of the tumor
- If the tumor involves the skull base, it usually does not invade the dura. The tumor can usually be dissected from the cranial dura with a clear dissection plane
- It should be noted that tumor with middle cranial fossa extension occasionally acquires a vascular supply from the middle meningeal artery and a tumor with anterior cranial fossa extension may have a vascular supply from the anterior and posterior ethmoidal arteries. If there is excessive bleeding from the surgery, a staged or combined open approach can be taken
- If there is a CSF leak, the tumor resection should proceed and skull base reconstruction can be performed later using an HBF

Once the tumor has been completely resected, the nasal cavity is irrigated with warm normal saline to control bleeding. Any further residual bleeding is controlled with bipolar cautery or temporary nasal packing.

Finally, Gelfoam (Pfizer, New York, NY, USA) is laid over areas of the nasopharynx, PPF and infratemporal fossa and pressure is applied using a Foley catheter for 48–72 hours.

Extended endoscopic approaches for malignant lesions

Extended endonasal endoscopic approaches (EEA) for excision of sinonasal malignant lesions are controversial but early experience reveals promising results (Nicolai et al. 2011). As a general oncological concept, the target of endoscopic surgery is radical removal of the lesion with negative margins confirmed by frozen section as in traditional open approaches. With an improved understanding of the endoscopic surgical anatomy and maturation in endoscopic surgical skills, together with extraordinary technological development, reconstruction of skull base defects after malignant tumor excision with vascularized flaps yield the most reliable outcomes with postoperative CSF leak rates of < 5% (Kassam et al. 2005).

Operative technique

- First, the nasal cavity is decongested with Moffat's solution (1 mL of adrenaline 1:1000, 2 mL of 10% cocaine, 4 mL of 8.4% sodium bicarbonate, 13 mL of water/saline) for 20 minutes
- Surgery commences with debulking of the intranasal portion of the tumor, assisted by a powered microdebrider or cutting instruments

with the intent to define the possible site of origin of the lesion and its relationship with the anterior skull base

- In most cases, these malignant lesions can be traced to a pedicle from where the tumor originates. The concept of endoscopic malignant tumor resection is to remove the tumor until the pedicle is identified and then remove the pedicle with a large margin of normal tissue confirmed by frozen section
- The 'dancing tumor' concept is very important in differentiating pedunculated tumor from tumor that has infiltrated surrounding structures. If the tumor is 'fixed' and not 'dancing' with the microdebrider, the surrounding structures should also be removed until normal tissue margins are obtained
- Debriding 'inside out,' starting at the core of the tumor, enables the capsules to collapse inward and this helps to identify areas of attachment to surrounding tissues (**Figure 13.6**)
- Malignant tumors tend to bleed and the bleeding will not stop until all of the tumor has been removed. Packing or bipolar diathermy of the bleeding surface to stop bleeding from a partially removed tumor may not be effective as all the raw tumor areas will continue to ooze. It is preferable to debride and remove as much tumor as quickly as possible and only to pack temporarily if there is so much bleeding that endoscopic vision is disrupted
- Whenever possible, try to identify and ligate or cauterize the feeding vessel(s) of the tumor
- With the magnifying power of endoscopes, the margins of resection are better defined. Any possible extension of the tumor should be excised and the negative margins confirmed by frozen section. This may include the posterior wall of the frontal sinus, anterior skull base, the medial wall of the orbit, the roof of the sphenoid sinus, and the nasal septum

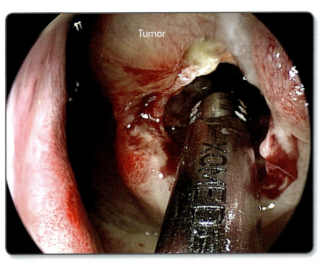

Figure 13.6 Endoscopic view of microdebrider debulking of a nasal tumor, using the concept of 'inside out' removal to allow the tumor to collapse in on itself.

- If the tumor has involved the bony anterior skull base, this bone is removed to expose any area of dural invasion. This is assisted by using a skull base drill. Bone removal can be extended from the crista galli to the planum sphenoidale and to the medial orbits bilaterally. The dura is then cauterized and incised lateral to the tumor. In esthesioneuroblastoma, the involved olfactory bulb and tract are also excised
- After completion of tumor excision, the next step is reconstruction of any skull base defect. Reconstruction with a pedicled nasoseptal HBF is the preferred choice if there is no compromise in the harvesting of the flap. This flap is useful to reconstruct defects located anywhere between from posterior wall of the frontal sinus to the lower clivus. It is always harvested at the start of the surgery to protect its pedicle
- A multilayer technique of reconstruction of skull base defects is preferred. An inlay subdural graft of collagen matrix is used to control the flow of the CSF. Subsequently, the nasoseptal flap is applied over the defect. Abdominal fat may be used to obliterate the dead space or the sphenoid sinus when appropriate. A biological glue can also be employed to anchor the flap
- Subsequently, nasal packing with the balloon of a 12-French Foley catheter is inserted under direct endoscopic visualization to bolster the flap against the defect for 48–72 hours

Postoperative care

- A broad-spectrum antibiotic is used until the nasal packing is removed after 48–72 hours
- A postoperative CT scan within the first 24 hours after surgery is routinely performed to rule out the presence of intracranial bleeding, parenchymal injury, and tension pneumocephalus
- The patient is advised to avoid excessive nose blowing, to sneeze and cough with an open mouth, to avoid any activities that may increase intracranial pressure such as abdominal straining, leaning forward and lifting anything heavier than 15 lb; and avoid using a tight collar
- The patient is given stool softeners to prevent straining and constipation
- The patient is taught how to perform nasal douching with saline solution
- The resulting surgical cavity is monitored endoscopically regularly in the outpatient clinic and debrided as needed. Interval CT and MRI scans are also undertaken depending on the extent of surgery and histological nature of the tumor

References

Batra PS, Citardi MJ, Worley S, et al. Resection of anterior skull base tumours: comparison of combined of combined traditional and endoscopic techniques. Am J Rhinol 2005; 19:521–8.

Doshi J, Youngs R. Navigational systems in rhinology – should we all be using them? J Laryngol Otol 2007; 121:818–21.

Hackman T, Snyderman CH, Carrau RL, Vescan A, Kassam A. Juvenile nasopharyngeal angiofibroma: the expanded endonasal approach. Am J Rhinol Allergy 2009; 23:95–9.

Hadad G, Bassagasteguy L, Carrau RL, et al. A novel reconstructive technique after endoscopic expanded endonasal approaches: vascular pedicle nasoseptal flap. Laryngoscope 2006; 116:1882–6.

Kassam AB, Carrau RL, Snyderman CH, Gardner P, Mintz A. Evolution of reconstructive techniques following endoscopic expanded endonasal approach. Neurosurg Focus 2005; 19:E8.

Lawson W, Patel ZM. The evolution of management for inverted papilloma: an analysis of 200 cases. Otolaryngol Head Neck Surg 2009; 140:330–35.

Luong A, Citardi MJ, Batra PS. Management of sinonasal malignant neoplasms: defining the role of endoscopy. Am J Rhino Allergy 2010; 24:150–5.

Maroldi R, Farina D, Battaglia G, et al. MR of malignant nasosinual neoplasms: frequently asked questions. Eur J Radiol 1997; 24:181–90.

Nicolai P, Castelnuovo P, Bolzoni Villaret A. Endoscopic resection of sinonasal malignancies. Curr Oncol Rep 2011; 13:138–44.

Ramakrishnan VR, Suh JD, Chiu AG, Palmer JN. Septal dislocation for access of the anterolateral maxillary sinus and infratemporal fossa. Am J Rhinol Allergy 2011; 25:128–30.

Zanation AM, Mitchell CA, Rose AS. Endoscopic skull base techniques for juvenile nasopharyngeal angiofibroma. Otolaryngol Clin North Am 2012; 45:711–30.

14 Glossectomy

Nicholas Stafford

Glossectomy is the removal of part or all of the tongue. If one lingual artery and the ipsilateral hypoglossal nerve can be preserved with a significant volume of anterior tongue musculature and mucosa then postoperative speech and swallowing may be impaired but should be acceptable. Significant difficulties with these crucial physiological functions occur when:

- Both lingual arteries are resected: the tongue bulk is likely to infarct and necrose
- Both hypoglossal nerves are damaged or divided: An immobile tongue is functionally useless
- Significant tongue base bulk is resected, even if one side is left intact: This is particularly true in the elderly who compensate badly
- There is significant tethering of the tongue, which can be caused by the use of insufficient tissue to close the defect. Paradoxically, using too bulky a reconstruction can have the same effect by reducing mobility of the residual mobile tongue
- A tongue base defect is reconstructed with a pedicled or free skin flap which is anesthetic. This will result in poor control of the food bolus

If a non-functioning 'tongue' is the likely result of surgery then the patient should be warned of the practical consequences which include the following:

- Inability to clear saliva and food from the oral cavity which can result in chronic dribbling
- Inability to articulate causing poorly comprehensible speech
- Inability to control the delivery of fluids and food into the pharynx resulting in a poorly co-ordinated swallow and the risk of overspill and consequent aspiration

Preoperative considerations

Broadly speaking, removal of half, or less than half of the anterior mobile tongue results in acceptable morbidity and can be tolerated well. However, if more than half of the tongue requires resection then non-surgical treatment should be considered as a better option particularly in terms of long-term morbidity. This is particularly true in the elderly who tend to compensate less well in response to loss of tongue musculature than do younger patients.

Total glossectomy is very rarely justified and should be reserved for those patients where:

- It is oncologically sound and is the only means of offering likely long-term survival
- The patient accepts that their postoperative speech and swallowing are going to be severely impaired
- The patient accepts that chronic overspill may necessitate a secondary laryngectomy just to secure a safe airway

A formal upper aerodigestive tract endoscopy, with biopsy of the primary tumor, is mandatory. Careful palpation of the tumor may demonstrate far greater extension into adjacent tissues than is appreciated visually. Does the tumor cross the midline?

For deeply seated tongue base tumors a tru-cut biopsy can be very helpful.

An MRI provides more information than CT with regard to soft tissue involvement and nodal metastases. In advanced stage disease PET–CT will help exclude the presence of distant metastases.

T1 and T2 tumors of the mobile tongue are best dealt with surgically and will seldom require planned postoperative radiotherapy. However, the latter will often be necessary for T3–T4 anterior tongue tumors and there is a good argument for treating such lesions with primary chemoradiotherapy – many such patients will be human papilloma virus (HPV) positive and therefore highly sensitive to these modalities. Radical surgery can be held in reserve for radioresistant or recurrent tumors.

If it is thought that primary surgery or chemoradiotherapy are likely to significantly impair swallowing during the treatment period and recovery phase, then a gastrostomy should be considered at the outset. It provides a guaranteed way of maintaining a good nutritional input and thereby body weight.

Staging

T1: < 2 cm in greatest diameter, and limited to mouth and/or oropharynx

T2: Between 2 cm and 4 cm in greatest diameter and linked to mouth and/or oropharynx

T3: > 4 cm in greatest diameter and limited to mouth and/or oropharynx

T4a: The tumor extends outside the contours of the tongue into immediately adjacent soft tissues, muscle or bone

T4b: The tumor extends to involve the pterygoid musculature, skull base or parapharyngeal space

For the reasons outlined above, surgery should only be used under exceptional circumstances for tumors of the tongue base. Many such tumors will be HPV positive and will probably be curable using chemoradiotherapy alone.

Partial glossectomy

As with any intraoral surgery, good access is essential. A nasal, as opposed to an oral, endotracheal tube is preferable. Where a significant portion of the tongue is to be resected and/or a flap reconstruction of the defect undertaken, then a temporary tracheostomy should be considered. A nasogastric tube (NGT) is passed at the time of the initial intubation.

A formal neck dissection should be undertaken for overt neck disease. A prophylactic level 1–3 or 2–5 conservative dissection (depending on the precise site of the primary) should be undertaken for the clinically and radiologically negative neck unless the primary is < 1 cm diameter and is superficial.

In practice, a hand held needle-point diathermy or CO_2 laser is best used for the dissection. Antibiotics are not routinely necessary, unless there is potential for bacterial contamination of the neck.

A Jennings mouth gag or rubber dental blocks are used to keep the mouth open. Through-and-through silk stitches can be used through the tongue tip to stabilize the tongue and allow better orientation with regard to the extent of the planned excision.

The anterior tongue

Tumors of the lateral border

- Use two silk stay sutures to immobilize the tongue (**Figure 14.1**) which is pulled forward in the midline
- The tumor is palpated and the proposed excision marked out using the diathermy or laser
- A macroscopic margin of 1–2 cm normal tissue around the tumor should be achieved with the dissection.
- Dissection commences anteriorly at the tongue tip
- Separation of the specimen from the residual tongue mass continues posteriorly through the tongue down to the frenum
- The inferior resection line extends posteriorly between the mobile tongue and floor of mouth: as much of the mucosa of the latter should be retained as is oncologically permissible
- Care should be taken not to breach the midline unless this is essential oncologically. If it is, make every effort to avoid damage to the contralateral lingual artery and hypoglossal nerve
- Continue the dissection as far posteriorly as is necessary. For a formal hemiglossectomy, use the circumvallate papillae as the posterior extent of the dissection
- Take the dorsal incision laterally to the lateral border of the tongue at or just behind junction of its anterior two thirds and posterior one third
- As the deeper musculature of the tongue is divided posteriorly the lingual artery will be encountered. This will require clipping and tying off

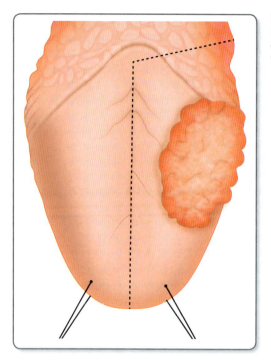

Figure 14.1 Two silk stay sutures are used to immobilize the tongue and dissection (following dashed line) commences anteriorly at the tongue tip.

- The entire specimen can then be dissected free and orientated using indicator ties for the benefit of the pathologist
- For a hemiglossectomy or anything less, a reconstruction using a pedicled or free flap is rarely necessary. As long as the adjacent floor of mouth has not been resected, the exposed tongue muscle can be left to re-epithelialize, although it is acceptable to directly close the anterior 3 cm using interrupted sutures
- Do not attempt to close the posterior part of the defect, as this will result in significant tethering of the tongue
- A quilted split skin graft can be used to cover the posterior part of the defect but only a limited 'take' is likely. It usually just provides a physiological dressing

A lateral tongue tumor will frequently extend inferiorly to involve the floor of the mouth and the management of such tumors will need to incorporate the principles of treatment of floor of mouth cancers as discussed in Chapter 15. The fate of the mandible is a crucial issue with regard to how such tumors are managed.

Tumors of the tongue tip or midline dorsum

- The resection margins for a tongue tip tumor are shown in **Figure 14.2**
- Primary closure of the resulting defect should be accomplished anteroposteriorly in order to retain as much tongue tip mobility as possible

For tumors of the midline dorsum, the best approach is to split the tongue in the midline, from the tip backward. The tumor can then be

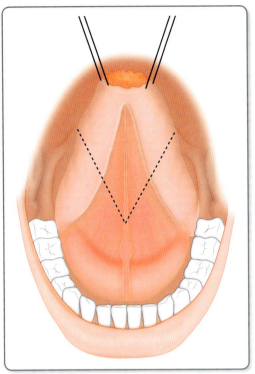

Figure 14.2 Resection margins for a tongue tip tumor.

approached directly and removed with an adequate margin. Avoid damage to the lingual arteries and hypoglossal nerves. Close the defect and the anterior tips using interrupted Vicryl sutures.

Surgical approach to larger tumors

Although the 'pull through' technique can be employed for some of these tumors, it is rarely the preferred option. However, it does have a role in terms of access for a total glossectomy, necessitating resection of the tongue base (see Chapter 9). Its chief advantage is the avoidance of splitting the mandible.

Any defect that is continuous with a neck dissection or which involves resection of more than half the tongue requires surgical reconstruction:

- A free skin flap has the advantage that certain types can be raised with a piece of bone for reconstruction of a mandibular defect. Free flaps should not be too bulky, but permit good mobility of the residual tongue
- Part of the function of the mobile tongue is to clear food and secretions from the oral cavity into the oropharynx: if it is likely that mobility of the residual tongue will be poor, then a more bulky myocutaneous flap should be considered (this can be free or pedicled). Filling the space left by the excised tongue will overcome the problem of an anterior floor of mouth sump effect where food and saliva accumulate and drooling becomes problematic

Careful postoperative assessment of the patients swallowing capabilities is essential. Oral feeding should not be commenced without an initial contrast swallow, which will provide information about the integrity of the mucosal closure and the risk of overspill and aspiration. Some patients will take weeks to rehabilitate and some will never do so. A few may even require a laryngectomy to protect their airway from chronic aspiration:

- If the tumor involving the anterior two-thirds and/or posterior third but does not impinge on the anterior mandibular arch then a lip split and midline mandibulotomy provide good surgical access
- A neck dissection incision is extended anteriorly and superiorly to split the lower lip (**Figure 14.3**)
- The bony mentum of the mandible is exposed for 1.5 cm each side of the midline, taking care to avoid damage to the mental nerves
- Before undertaking a stepped mandibulotomy, mark out the planned osteotomy and drill the appropriate holes for the plates to be used to reoppose the two halves of the mandible. This makes subsequent closure easier and more accurate
- The mandibulotomy is made using an oscillating saw
- Using retractors, the two halves of the mandible are retracted laterally, like opening the covers of a book
- Good access to the oral cavity is provided and excision of the tumor undertaken safely with good exposure of local anatomy
- Use stay sutures, as before, to stabilize the tongue and help preserve normal anatomical relationships (**Figure 14.4**)

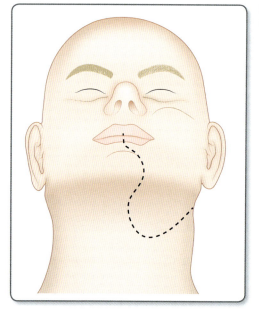

Figure 14.3 Neck dissection incision extended anteriorly and superiorly to split the lower lip.

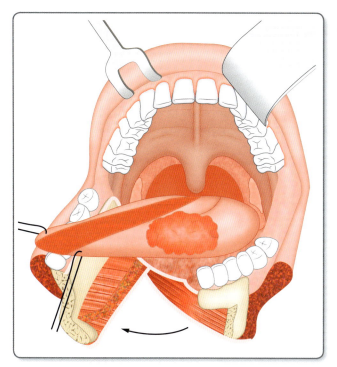

Figure 14.4 Using retractors, the two halves of the mandible are retracted laterally, allowing good access to the oral cavity and safe excision of the tumor with good exposure of local anatomy. Stay sutures stabilize the tongue and help preserve normal anatomical relationships.

- Palpation of the tumor is helpful is securing adequate excision margins. Frozen sections can be used as appropriate
- Without compromising oncological principles, make every attempt to preserve at least one lingual artery and hypoglossal nerve

Tumor involvement of the mandible necessitates either a marginal or segmental mandibulectomy. If the tumor is anterior and crosses the midline, then the surgical approach described above can be used. Alternatively a visor approach, not splitting the lip, can be adopted though this will result in an anesthetic lower lip (to be avoided unless necessary for adequate tumor clearance) (see Chapter 9 for details).

For lateralized tumors a lateral approach is employed:

- Mobilize the superior flap of the neck dissection incision superiorly to provide adequate exposure of the mandible
- Skeletonize the lateral aspect of the mandible to allow good access
- Strip the periosteum off the bone at the sites of the two osteotomies
- Expose only as much of the bone of the lingual aspect of the mandible as is required for each osteotomy
- Remove any teeth that will interfere with execution of the osteotomies
- Use an oscillating saw for the bone cuts. Protect the intraoral mucosa using malleable retractors
- Undertake the intraoral part of the resection and remove the specimen en bloc

The role of a head and neck speech and language therapist is essential for the speech and swallowing rehabilitation of these patients. Two significant determinants of outcome are age and size of resection. It can take several weeks for the gastrostomy to become unnecessary, and in a minority of cases it will be a permanent requirement. Using videofluoroscopy and clinical assessment aspiration/overspill can be monitored. If this continues to be significant 10–12 weeks postsurgery then the option of a salvage laryngectomy needs to be considered.

Further reading

Huang SF, Kang CJ, Lun CY, et al. Neck treatment of patients with early stage oral tongue cancer: comparison between observation, supramohyoid dissection and extended dissection. Cancer 2008; 112:1066–75.

Kokemueller H, Rama M, Rubback J, et al. The Hanover experience: surgical treatment of tongue cancer – a clinical retrospective evaluation over a 30 year period. Head Neck Oncol 2011; 3:1–9.

15 Management of the mandible in squamous cell carcinoma of the oral cavity

Richard J. Shaw

The management of the mandible is one of the most frequent dilemmas in planning treatment for oral malignancy. Tumors frequently present adjacent to, or invading, the mandible and the requirement for clear bone and soft tissue margins often dictates some form of mandibular resection. It is known that the subsites of oral cancer do not have differing prognosis, provided they are competently managed (Shaw et al. 2009), so functional and aesthetic outcomes are key.

Prior to the era of effective microvascular reconstruction, the devastating results of surgery were all too apparent and characterized as the 'Andy Gump' appearance. Historically, this situation was compounded by erroneous theories of bone invasion and similarly erroneous concerns about the periosteal path of lymphatic drainage, both resulting in the over utilization of oromandibular 'Commando' resections with poor reconstructions and little chance of functional rehabilitation (Brown 2003).

Because of the close proximity of the mandible to the commonest sites of oral squamous cell carcinoma (OSCC), itself the commonest form of head and neck squamous cell carcinoma (HNSCC), then careful preoperative staging (Brown & Lewis-Jones 2001, Brown 2003) and assessment is a crucial step in planning resections. Understanding the detailed requirements for reconstruction and rehabilitation (Shaw et al. 2005) of the mandibular defect is an essential prerequisite in planning surgery for OSCC. Specific skills in managing malignancy close to the mandible are an essential component of the head and neck multidisciplinary team.

Staging and workup

In addition to the usual diagnostic imaging and staging for OSCC, it is important to determine as accurately as possible whether the bone is invaded or not, and to what extent. This assessment is made in the context of:

- Position of the tumor
- MRI and CT assessment of tumor extent and bone invasion
- Biological behavior of the tumor
- Dental status
- Height of the mandible (which in edentulous patients, may be judged with the aid of the Cawood & Howell classification (Brown et al. 2005) (**Table 15.1**)

The underlying principle is that the mandible shows the greatest risk or degree of invasion at the closest point to the tumor. Previously, it has been theorized that preferential invasion through periodontium or mandibular foramen occurs but this has been effectively disproved by the evidence, and, put simply, the tumor invades where it touches the jaw. The relative merits of imaging to diagnose bone invasion (Brown & Lewis-Jones 2001) are shown in **Table 15.2**. Because no one method is completely accurate, some procedures must be undertaken with a range of surgical options available reflecting this uncertainty. Correspondingly, it is important to have made adequate assessment of all composite flap donor sites, have gained suitable consent and theatre time, even when they are not expected to be needed.

Surgical technique

Ablation

The underlying principles of surgery for OSCC involving the mandible are similar to any other resection of a malignant tumor, namely:

- Adequate access
- Resection with clear margins in three dimensions

Table 15.1 Guide to mandibular resection based on degree of invasion and degree of mandible resorption			
Cawood & Howell classification	OPT −ve, MRI −ve, Bone scan −ve, No invasion or only periosteal invasion	OPT −ve, MRI +ve, Bone scan +ve, Early invasion (< 5 mm)	OPT +ve, MRI +ve, Bone scan +ve Invasion > 5 mm
I–II (dentate or immediate postextension)	Rim	Rim	Rim or Segment
III–IV (round or knife edge)	Rim	Rim or segment	Segment
V–VI (flat or depressed ridge)	Rim or segment	Segment	Segment
MRI, magnetic resonance imaging; OPT, orthopantomogram.			

| Table 15.2 Accuracy of detecting mandibular invasion | | | |
	OPT (orthopantomogram)	MRI (magnetic resonance imaging)	Bone scan (3D SPECT)
Sensitivity	50%	66%	85%
Specificity	~100%	85%	85%

- Appropriate reconstruction to restore form and function

In locally advanced tumors close to the mandible, a tracheostomy is usually helpful to facilitate access and safe postoperative airway management. A tracheostomy is indicated with:

- Bilateral neck dissections
- Segmental resection
- Trismus
- Larger (>4 cm) tumors

Tumors of the floor of mouth have rather insubstantial anatomical barriers to invasion and as a result great care must be taken to ensure clear margins. Due to significant shrinkage of tissues on fixation, a deep intraoperative margin of 10–15 mm may be necessary to ensure pathologically 'clear' margins of 5 mm. This situation might be compared with, for example, glottic tumors where the cartilaginous skeleton of the larynx presents a more favorable environment in regards of both anatomical barriers and shrinkage. For this reason, de-escalation of surgery using laser excision that might be advocated in the larynx ('TORL') is recommended only for T1 and early T2 tumors in most oral cavity sites. Further, the deep extent of a larger tumor may invade through the floor of mouth structures, making a combined per-oral and cervical approach logical. The consequences of such defects regarding risk of orocutaneous fistula make free tissue transfer a necessary procedure to ensure speedy healing and prompt discharge.

However, the universal application of 'heroic' access procedures should be avoided, with their inherent scarring and frequent complications:

- Lip split and mandibulotomy are rarely needed unless tumors are posterior or there is severe trismus
- In segmental mandibular resection, good access is afforded after carrying out the osteotomies (without lip split), which should therefore be established as early as possible in the resection
- Avoid extensive lingual release ('visor') other than that specifically inherent in tumor resection, as this has been shown to cause severe swallowing dysfunction and increase the risk of orocutaneous fistula

In planning the resection of bone, the situation is self-evident when a mandible shows gross invasion (T4). In these cases, the complete height of mandible including lower border must be resected, termed a segmental resection. Following this a composite reconstruction is usually indicated. The position of the surrounding mandible must be secured with a prelocated spanning osteosynthesis plate or with intermaxillary fixation. Resection of the condyle is rarely needed in managing OSCC and retaining a substantial proximal fragment greatly facilitates mandibular reconstruction. The decision to retain the lower border of the mandible with a rim resection is fundamental in avoiding morbidity and the complexities of composite reconstruction. In many cases (**Figure 15.1a**), a dentate mandible might be at risk of invasion with a T2 adjacent floor of mouth tumor, however, if the tumor does not invade deeply, an obliquely angled rim resection (dotted line) is possible. This can be achieved without the need for composite reconstruction and surgery. In **Figure 15.1b**, it can be seen that a similar tumor in the context of a severely resorbed edentulous mandible requires a segmental resection. Similarly in **Figure 15.1c**, a dentate mandible may need composite resection, even with equivocal bone invasion if a larger tumor (T3/4) deeply invades the lingual tissue.

Where a shallow tumor shows equivocal invasion at the alveolus, it is often preferable to perform a 'defensive' rim resection. It should not be expected that 100% of rim or segmental resections will show frank invasion on the pathology report (Shaw et al. 2004a) as the surgeon does not have the diagnostic luxuries in the operating theatre afforded to the histopathologist. One method that can safely be applied to reduce the rate of negative bone resections is intraoperative periosteal stripping (Brown et al. 1994). Where a tumor is close but felt to be clear of bone, it is permissible to explore subperiosteally, under direct vision and where periosteum is intact, bone resection might be avoided. Similarly, where a rim resection is favored, the remaining periosteum can be checked after bony resection. In either case, where tumor is encountered, the tissues can be replaced and a more radical approach executed. In skilled hands, it is rare to find involved bone margins on final staging, and in such cases there is often a highly infiltrative pattern of invasion (Shaw et al. 2004a) and accompanying features of adverse prognosis such as involved soft tissue margins, extracapsular nodal disease and perineural invasion.

In the case of a deeper rim resection, it may be preferable to place a reconstruction plate in order to avoid the risk of pathological fracture

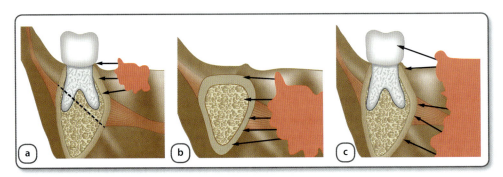

Figure 15.1 Influence of depth of invasion and height of mandible on resection type.

(although admittedly opinion differs on whether this eventually weakens the mandible through stress shielding) (**Figure 15.2**).

Reconstruction

The gold standard for segmental reconstruction following malignancy is for composite free flap reconstruction at the time of resection. This option has now replaced the use of alloplastic bridging plates and offers several critical advantages:

- Reduces need for further major surgery
- Takes advantage of vascular access at the time of neck dissection
- Avoids the difficulty of secondary repair of the defect after inevitable scarring has occurred
- With twin team operating, often flap harvest can be simultaneous with the ablative surgery
- Avoids healing complications that are near universal after irradiation of a bridging plate

The requirement for reconstruction is particularly evident in the anterior mandibular defect and in those patients retaining significant dentition. In smaller posterior defects with edentulous patients, then occasionally a compromise may be to leave a segment without reconstruction, particularly in the presence of severe comorbidity:

A few hints may be useful when planning reconstruction:

- Try to utilize the natural curvature of the bone flap to reduce the number of osteotomies needed
- Reconstruction of the anterior mandible is always more challenging than posterior segments, and poor results less well tolerated
- Try to use closing osteotomies if sufficient bone and pedicle length exists, otherwise opening osteotomies can be used to great effect if length inadequate
- It is often helpful in edentulous cases to slightly reduce the span of reconstructed mandible between resection and reconstruction to prevent class III appearance (approximately one- or two-screw holes)
- Avoid free bone if at all possible; these reliably become the nidus for persisting infection, made worse by the use of radiotherapy
- Although complications are similar between reconstruction plates and miniplate osteosynthesis (Shaw et al. 2004b), the former

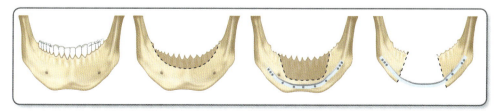

Figure 15.2 From L to R: mandible prior to resection; defensive rim resection; deep rim resection for invaded mandible reinforced with a reconstruction plate; segmental resection with prelocated unilock plate awaiting bone flap.

makes prelocation easier and the latter are easier to remove if they become infected
- Although the length of bone and pedicle are often cited as factors in choosing donor site, the average defect is 6–10 cm (Shaw et al. 2004b) and immediately adjacent to immediately availably neck vessels, so neither is often an issue
- Always have in mind an alternative donor site to allow for the rare event of flap failure, for example when choosing a site for an arterial line or skin graft. For the same reason think carefully about the need for a staged bilateral neck dissection

The choice of donor site is a much debated topic with many advocates for each technique. The underlying guiding principles are as follows:
1. To match the form and constituents of the resection and reconstruction
2. Avoid donor site morbidity
3. Avoid complications in the neomandible
4. Shorten operation time when possible
5. Facilitate implant based oral rehabilitation

The advantages and disadvantages of the four common donor sites (Shaw et al. 2004b) are tabulated in **Table 15.3** and shown in the annotated cases comprising **Figure 15.3**.

Rehabilitation

The details of oral rehabilitation are beyond the scope of this chapter but a few summary points are presented (Shaw et al. 2005):
- Few patients manage to retain teeth after treatment for oral cancers near the alveolus, and almost none manage to wear a conventional lower denture after surgery
- Many patients will gain great benefit as a result of oral rehabilitation based on osseointegrated implants
- Once a patient gains insight that they have been cured, their motivation for improving aesthetic and functional aspects is often surprisingly good
- Although many patients will not meet the conventional criteria for implants, the results in selected patients are generally excellent and longstanding
- The indications for placement of implants are reasonable prognosis, suitable motivation and adequate retention of oral function
- Implants can be inserted as a primary (at the time of resection) or a secondary (after completion of treatment) procedure
- It is key to involve a rehabilitation/prosthetics specialist at the time of treatment planning, and indefinitely following rehabilitation, in order to optimize the chances of success

Table 15.3 Relative merits of composite flap donor sites				
Donor site	Fibula	DCIA	Scapula	Composite RFFF
Donor site morbidity	++	++	+++	+
Pedicle length	+++	+	+	++++
Quality of vessels	+++/+ (frequently affected by atherosclerosis)	++ (may be quite small)	++++ (large) (unaffected by atherosclerosis)	+++ (unaffected by atherosclerosis)
Volume of bone	++	++++	+++	+
Length of bone	++++ (14 cm)	+++ (12 cm)	++ (10 cm)	+++ (12 cm)
Suitability for implants	+++	++++	+++	Unsuited
Soft tissue paddle	++ (occasionally unreliable)	++ (as either internal oblique, DCIA perf. flap)	+++ (allowing two soft tissue flaps and as a chimera with LD or TAP)	++ (although lacks bulk)
Two team operating	++++	+++	+	+++
DCIA, deep circumflex iliac artery; LD, latissimus dorsi; RFFF, radial forearm free flap; TAP, thoracodorsal artery perforator				

Complications

As in many aspects of head and neck surgery, medical complications are frequent and usually correlated more closely to the comorbidities the patient presents with, rather than age or magnitude of surgery. Flap failure is frequently rare in experienced hands (around 2–5%) and is similar between the various donor sites. Large resections run the risk of orocutaneous fistulae but these are usually self-limiting with effective free flap reconstructions.

Later complications are often related to the requirement for radiotherapy (Shaw et al. 2004b) in many patients. If irradiated, the majority of osteosynthesis plates become subject to chronic infection and require removal (Shaw et al. 2004b). Similarly, osteoradionecrosis will occur in 5–10% of long-term survivors who have had radiotherapy. Functional problems with speech and swallowing correlate more with the extent of soft tissue resection and need for adjuvant radiotherapy, provided the mandible is adequately managed. As these factors are largely predictable from careful staging, this is largely an issue for consent. A long-term gastrostomy and/or tracheostomy are generally avoidable.

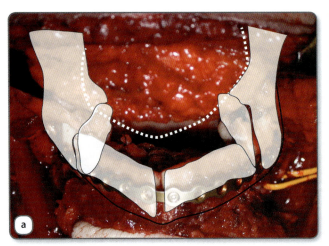

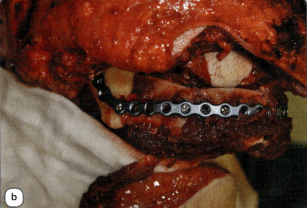

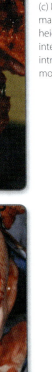

Figure 15.3 Examples of segmental reconstructions to reconstruct anterior mandibular defect. (a) Fibula: Although satisfactory and implantable, this shallow strut of bone often results in a quite a shrunken appearance to the lower third of the face after radiotherapy. The fibula's profile only allows reconstruction equivalent to a severely resorbed mandible unless used as a 'double-barrel'. (b) Scapula: Good height is available, an often quite adequate length. In this case combined with both parascapular and thoracodorsal artery perforator flaps to allow both intra- and extraoral soft tissue reconstruction which is a particularly versatile feature of the subscapular system. (c) DCIA to reconstruct anterior mandibular defect gives excellent height and width, in this case the internal oblique will be reflected intraorally to reconstruct the floor of mouth. *Contd...*

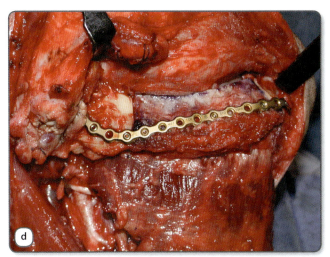

Figure 15.3 *Contd...* (d) Another DCIA, but in this case an anterior and lateral combined defect – note that the natural curvature of the iliac crest allows it to be satisfactorily inset without an osteotomy.

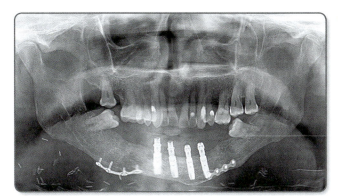

Figure 15.4 Osseointegrated implants placed in a scapula flap at the anterior mandible.

References

Brown J. Mechanisms of cancer invasion of the mandible. Curr Opin Otolaryngol Head Neck Surg 2003; 11:96–102.

Brown J, Chatterjee R, Lowe D, et al. A new guide to mandibular resection for oral squamous cell carcinoma based on the Cawood and Howell classification of the mandible. Int J Oral Maxillofac Surg 2005; 34:834–9.

Brown JS, Griffith JF, Phelps PD, et al. A comparison of different imaging modalities and direct inspection after periosteal stripping in predicting the invasion of the mandible by oral squamous cell carcinoma. Br J Oral Maxillofac Surg 1994; 32:347–59.

Brown JS, Lewis-Jones H. Evidence for imaging the mandible in the management of oral squamous cell carcinoma: a review. Br J Oral Maxillofac Surg 2001; 39:411–8.

Shaw RJ, Brown JS, Woolgar JA, et al. The influence of the pattern of mandibular invasion on recurrence and survival in oral squamous cell carcinoma. Head Neck 2004; 26:861–9.

Shaw RJ, Kanatas AN, Lowe D, et al. Comparison of miniplates and reconstruction plates in mandibular reconstruction. Head Neck 2004; 26:456–63.

Shaw RJ, McGlashan G, Woolgar JA, et al. Prognostic importance of site in squamous cell carcinoma of the buccal mucosa. Br J Oral Maxillofac Surg 2009; 47:356–9.

Shaw RJ, Sutton AF, Cawood JI, et al. Oral rehabilitation after treatment for head and neck malignancy. Head Neck 2005; 27:459–70.

16 Parotid cancer

Terry M. Jones

Cancer of the major salivary glands is rare, occurring at an incidence of 8–9 per million population per year. While the parotid is the most common site for a salivary gland neoplasm most are benign. This is in contrast to neoplasms of the submandibular, sublingual or minor salivary glands, which are more likely to be malignant. They are rare in patients younger than 50 years of age and malignant tumors have an equal gender distribution.

Neoplasms of the parotid (and other salivary glands) constitute a heterogeneous group of tumors presenting with variable histopathological features – which ensure that diagnosis may be challenging. Common malignant tumors of the salivary gland, as recognized by the WHO, are listed in **Table 16.1**. Typically, tumors are reported as histologically high, low or mixed grade – the latter classification indicating variable clinical behavior depending on the relative abundance of distinct, biologically variable, histological features. However, this histological grading system has proved unreliable for all tumors apart from mucoepidermoid carcinoma, to the point that clinical features and behavior should be relied upon more when deciding upon treatment stratagems.

Staging

T staging for major salivary gland tumors is as set out in the UICC version 7, which is outlined in **Table 16.2**.

Clinical presentation

Almost invariably, parotid cancer presents as a mass in the parotid gland (**Figure 16.1**). Usually the mass is evident under the skin of the face, indicating the presence of the tumor in, at least, the superficial lobe of the parotid gland. While the mass could emanate from any area

Table 16.1 WHO classification of malignant salivary gland tumors 2005	
Malignant epithelial tumors	**Hematolymphoid tumors**
Acinic cell carcinoma	Hodgkin lymphoma
Mucoepidermoid carcinoma	Metastasizing pleomorphic adenoma
Adenoid cystic carcinoma	Diffuse large B-cell lymphoma
Polymorphous low-grade adenocarcinoma	Extranodal marginal zone B cell lymphoma
Epithelial myoepithelial carcinoma	
Clear cell carcinoma, not otherwise specified	
Basal cell adenocarcinoma	
Sebaceous carcinoma	
Sebaceous lymphadenocarcinoma	
Cystadenocarcinoma	
Low-grade cribriform cystadenocarcinoma	
Mucinous adenocarcinoma	
Oncocytic carcinoma	
Salivary duct carcinoma	
Squamous cell carcinoma	
Undifferentiated carcinoma	
Small cell carcinoma	
Large cell carcinoma	
Lymphoepithelial carcinoma	
Adenocarcinoma, not otherwise specified	
Carcinoma ex pleomorphic adenoma malignant mixed tumor	
Myoepithelial carcinoma	

Table 16.2 T staging for major salivary gland tumors is as set out in the (UICC version 7)	
T stage	**Primary tumor cannot be assessed**
T0	No evidence of primary tumor
T1	Tumor ≤ 2 cm in greatest dimension without extraparenchymal extension*
T2	Tumor > 2 cm but ≤ 4 cm in greatest dimension without extraparenchymal extension*
T3	Tumor > 4 cm and/or tumor having extraparenchymal extension*
T4a	Tumor invades skin, mandible, ear canal, and/or facial nerve
T4b	Tumor invades skull base and/or pterygoid plates and/or encases carotid artery

*Extraparenchymal extension is clinical or macroscopic evidence of invasion of soft tissues. Microscopic evidence alone does not constitute extraparenchymal extension for classification purposes.

of the parotid gland, masses are most common in the inferior or caudal regions of the gland. Deep lobe tumors may present as asymmetric swellings of the parapharynx. Often these are discovered incidentally following throat examination for other reasons, or the patient may experience a sensation of fullness or even present with apparently unrelated symptoms such as enhanced snoring or ipsilateral nasal obstruction. Usually such masses are slow growing, but rapid expansion can occur especially in the case of carcinoma ex-pleomorphic salivary adenoma (PSA) or lymphoma. In the case of rapidly expanding tumors it is not unusual for the tumor to have already involved overlying skin. In this case, curative treatment is likely to be less successful and reconstruction would need to be considered in light of the necessity to resect skin during surgery.

In all cases of parotid cancer, spread to the regional lymph nodes may, or may not be, clinically evident and so the role of a neck dissection needs to be considered on the merits of each case.

Diagnosis

Clinical examination

Following the taking of an appropriate history, a full head and neck examination should be completed. The mass should be palpated to establish its clinical consistency and local extent.

Even in the case of an apparent superficial lobe tumor, a careful examination of the oropharynx should be undertaken in an attempt to establish any deep lobe extension that would result in the presence of a mass deep to the tonsil with consequent medial displacement. If oro- or nasopharyngeal asymmetry is detected, a flexible, fiberoptic nasendoscopic examination would be advisable in an attempt to establish the cranial extent of the mass.

Ultrasound-guided fine needle aspiration cytology

Ultrasound-guided fine needle aspiration cytology (USS FNAC) is often a key to the diagnosis of a malignant parotid tumor and most people would agree that it is mandatory. However, the technique does have limits with respect to sensitivity and specificity, which relate:

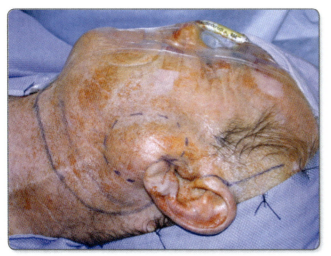

Figure 16.1 Standard draping and pre-operative preparation of a patient undergoing surgery for a malignant left parotid mass. The mass is circumscribed by a broken line and the planned skin incision is indicated by a continuous line.

1. To the technical limitation of the technique itself and the subsequent histological diagnosis of the cytological specimen (which appears to be very operator dependent)
2. To the heterogeneous nature of parotid neoplasms

It follows that the false negative rate of FNAC in the diagnosis of parotid cancer is not insignificant and negative results should be treated with caution and correlated closely with the clinical picture

Preoperative investigation

All cases of parotid cancer should be discussed by the regional head and neck cancer multidisciplinary team (MDT) in order to achieve consensus with respect to treatment offered.

Most clinicians advocate preoperative imaging as guided by the protocols laid down by the local head and neck cancer MDT, but in most cases this will involve ultrasound scanning, MR, or CT imaging of the head and neck with CT imaging of the thorax and upper abdomen. The latter is particularly important when the primary diagnosis is of a tumor known to have significant metastatic potential, e.g. adenoid cystic carcinoma.

The appearance seen on imaging – whatever modality is used – can be predictive of malignant potential, which may be of particular significance if there is ambiguity surrounding FNAC diagnosis.

Treatment options

Surgery followed by adjuvant external beam radiotherapy is the mainstay of treatment for parotid cancer.

Perioperative antibiotics should not be routinely given.

Consent to surgical treatment

The following points should be raised when consenting all patients undergoing surgery for parotid cancer:

- The need to create a surgical wound that would result in an inevitable scar and the small risk of postoperative infection and hematoma that might require further surgical intervention
- Additional consent relating to reconstruction would need to be sought if the surgical extirpation of the tumor also required excision of overlying skin
- Damage to branches of the facial nerve that may be permanent
- Paraesthesia in the distribution of the great auricular nerve
- Gustatory sweating in the distribution of the facial nerve (Frey's syndrome)
- Postoperative salivary fistula and its consequences
- The potential need for adjuvant non-surgical treatment
- The expected prognosis depending upon the definitive histopathology report

Incisions

Conventionally, a Modified Blair, or 'Lazy S' incision is advocated for parotid surgery. It is usual during surgery for parotid cancer to ensure that the inferior, cervical limb of this incision is placed to facilitate adequate exposure for the completion of a neck dissection, should this be planned or anticipated (**Figure 16.2**). Even if a neck dissection is not undertaken, positioning of the cervical limb in this way allows greater exposure to the structures of the upper neck that will make identification of the facial nerve trunk easier. If cosmesis is an issue to consider, the upper aspect of the incision can be continued behind the tragus rather than in front. While modified facelift incisions have been advocated for benign parotid surgery in an attempt to improve cosmesis from scar formation, this approach is often contraindicated in all but the most experienced surgical hands when undertaking surgery for parotid cancer as surgical exposure is markedly reduced.

Operative technique

Preparation

- During surgery the patient is placed in a supine position with the cervical spine extended at C6/7 by a cushion placed under the patient's shoulders and the head of the operating table extended. Additional exposure is often achieved by rotating the patient's head away from the side of the procedure
- Standard skin preparation is undertaken and the patient is draped to allow adequate exposure of the surgical field. The author finds it helpful to drape the face of the patient with a transparent cellophane dressing to allow visualization of the ipsilateral face while maintaining surgical sterility (Figure 16.1)
- Many surgeons advocate the use a facial nerve monitor during surgery, in an attempt to minimize the likelihood of facial nerve damage. Others, including the author, find the use of a facial nerve

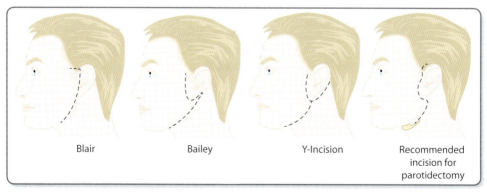

Blair   Bailey   Y-Incision   Recommended
                                                    incision for
                                                    parotidectomy

Figure 16.2 Commonly used incision for parotid gland tumor surgery (far right).

monitor an irritation during parotid surgery as the monitor is often activated when surgery is taking place some distance from important branches of the facial nerve

- Subcutaneous infiltration of 1/200,000 adrenaline to the area overlying the parotid gland may be employed in an attempt to minimize bleeding while raising the surgical skin flaps

Exposing the facial nerve

- Following incision of the skin and subcutaneous tissues, skin flaps are developed to allow access to the parotid gland and the structures of the neck. Over the face the flap is developed deep to the submuscular aponeuritic system (SMAS) layer, while in the neck a standard subplatysmal flap is developed
- The skin flaps are developed to allow visualization of the entire parotid gland and at least lymph node levels I and II of the neck, even when a formal neck dissection is not planned. Should a neck dissection be planned, then wider exposure of the neck will be required
- It is the author's preference to aim for maximal surgical exposure of the structures associated with identification of the facial nerve trunk in an attempt to avoid searching for the nerve trunk down 'a deep dark hole.' This involves starting inferiorly to identify the posterior belly of the digastric (PBD) muscle. Following this muscle belly in a craniodorsal direction – which is technically extremely easy – leads to the insertion of the muscle in the digastric notch on the deep surface of the mastoid portion of the temporal bone. The facial nerve trunk emerges deep to the PBD through the stylomastoid foramen and so is always protected as long as dissection is continued lateral to the PBD. This dissection of the PBD also leads to good exposure of the posterior and posteroinferior borders of the parotid gland
- Next, the tragal cartilage is identified and used as a marker to facilitate dissection in a cranial and caudal direction along the posterior, or dorsal, edge of the parotid gland. As the dissection proceeds the dorsal edge of the parotid gland is retracted forward to maximize exposure. During this dissection, the tragal pointer – the spear-like projection of the deep aspect of the tragal cartilage – and the tympanomastoid suture are easily identified
- The approach to the facial nerve trunk from an inferior and superior direction along a broad front ensures wide exposure of the entire dorsal aspect of the parotid gland and facilitates the easy and safe identification of the three structures – the tragal pointer, the tympanomastoid suture and the PBD – necessary for the safe identification of the facial nerve trunk
- The facial nerve trunk is then identified by deeper dissection following the tympanomastoid suture between the tragal pointer and the PBD
- Once identified, a nerve stimulator can be used to confirm correct identification of the facial nerve

Facial nerve dissection

- In cases where the tumor is large and/or overlying the trunk of the facial nerve, it may be advantageous to identify the branches of the nerve by retrograde dissection. This technique requires identification of the terminal branches of the facial nerve, as they exit the anterior border of the gland. Retrograde dissection along individual branches, toward the main trunk, then proceeds using the techniques outlined below
- A mosquito clip is used for careful dissection along the superficial surface of the facial nerve trunk. This maneuver creates a 'tunnel' of parotid tissue over the surface of the nerve, which can be increased in size by gently retraction of the open jaws of the clip superficially allowing better visualization of the distal portions of the nerve (**Figure 16.3**)
- The elevated parotid tissue is then incised following bipolar diathermy coagulation, thereby exposing the portion of the nerve deep to the incision line. (The author prefers to use a curved No. 12 scalpel blade for incising the elevated parotid tissue). The maneuver is then repeated as often as required to allow full exposure of the facial nerve and its constituent trunks
- It is important to note that the exact progress and direction of facial nerve exposure will be governed by the direction and branching pattern of the branches of the nerve as well as the position of the tumor within the parotid gland, accepting that it is oncologically essential to ensure the maximum possible normal tissue margin around the tumor
- During surgery for parotid cancer it is not unusual to have to resect parts of, or the entire, deep lobe of the parotid gland. In this case, the nerve is initially identified and exposed as above. Following this, individual branches of the nerve are dissected free so that they can be retracted superiorly or inferiorly to allow access to the deep lobe of the gland. During resection of the deep lobe it is essential to identify the retromandibular vein and external carotid artery that

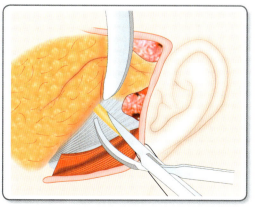

Figure 16.3 Recommended technique for resecting parotid tissue and/or tumor while protecting the facial nerve.

are embedded within the gland, deep to the facial nerve, in order to clip and tie them

Post-resection

- In parotid cancer surgery there is often debate about the relative merits of sacrificing the facial nerve during surgery. Most surgeons now subscribe to the view that if the nerve is working prior to surgery, all efforts should be taken to preserve all branches of the nerve as long as macroscopic residual tumor is not left adherent to it. The evidence suggests that sacrificing the nerve branches confers no survival advantage but markedly reduces quality of life. This rationale is irrelevant if there is pre-existing facial nerve paralysis. In this case, the relevant branches should be resected along with the tumor. Whatever the circumstances of facial nerve branch resection, facial nerve reconstruction, using, for example, great auricular nerve cable grafts, should be considered in the context of the individual case, although functional results are frequently disappointing
- Following resection of the tumor, depending on the size of the surgical defect, drains may be placed in situ. If suction drains are to be used, care should be taken to ensure that the drain is situated distant from the nerve to avoid suction trauma
- Thrombin-based tissue glues may be used to enhance repositioning of the skin flaps and reduce the risk of postoperative hematoma and the surgical wound is closed using a layer of subcutaneous absorbable sutures to reoppose the SMAS and platysmal layers and an appropriate skin suture. (The author prefers to use subcuticular-beaded proline in an attempt to optimize the cosmetic appearance of the surgical scar.)
- Drains are removed when they collect < 20 mL of transudate in 24 hours and, in the absence of complications, the patient is discharged

Postoperative complications

The most common postoperative complications have been listed as part of the section on preoperative consent above. Should any postoperative complication occur, it should be managed according to the merits of the specific case.

The most commonly occurring complications include facial nerve paresis or paralysis and salivary fistula.

In the case of the former, initial management is conservative and should include measures to minimize corneal scarring if the patient is unable to actively close the eye. This often involves the use of lubricant eye gels as required and – particularly during sleep – taping of the eyelid to ensure eye closure is also often advised. More definitive solutions for facial nerve paralysis include a variety of surgical static and dynamic facial reanimation procedures. Whether they are employed depends on the merits of each individual case.

Salivary fistula results from the continued secretion of saliva from the cut surface of the parotid gland deep to the skin flap. Initially a collection of saliva occurs (sialocele) before the saliva finds the line of least resistance to drain transcutaneously usually via the surgical scar. Initial management is conservative when pressure dressings and frequent aspiration of the sialocele may be undertaken. Anticholinergic drugs may be prescribed in an attempt to reduce saliva flow but their use is often limited by their attendant troublesome side effects. In contrast, botulinum toxin, injected into the gland, exerts its effect locally by enhancing the proteasomal degradation of SNAP-25 – a protein required for vesicle formation and the release of neurotransmitters (including acetylcholine) from axonal endings – and its use is therefore not limited by debilitating systemic side effects. In rare resistant cases radiotherapy, tympanic nerve section and even total parotidectomy have been recommended with varying levels of success.

Further reading

Drake R, Vogl AW, Mitchell AWM. Gray's Anatomy for Students, 2nd edn. Philadelphia, PA: Churchill Livingstone, 2009.

Shah JP, Patel SG, Singh B. Jatin Shah's Head and Neck Surgery and Oncology, 4th edn. Philadelphia, PA: Mosby Elsevier, 2012.

Witt RL. Salivary Gland Diseases: Surgical and Medical Management. New York: Thieme, 2005.

Surgery of the infratemporal fossa and adjacent skull base

Tristram Lesser

Surgery of the infratemporal fossa and skull base is indicated for the following:

1. The removal of tumors involving the skull base, e.g. glomus jugulare tumors, chordomas, temporal bone cancers, and olfactory neuroblastomas
2. To provide access to the intracranial cavity, e.g. for petroclival meningiomas and vestibular schwannomas
3. To enable removal of head and neck malignancies which have spread medially and superiorly to involve the skull base, e.g. parotid or sinus cancers

Anatomy of the infratemporal fossa

Surgery of the infratemporal fossa remains the key to all skull base surgery except for lesions limited to the midline. A good understanding of its complex three-dimensional anatomy is essential.

Principles of infratemporal fossa and skull base surgery

The infratemporal fossa is a potential space inferior to the temporal bone and the greater wing of the sphenoid. It is lateral to the pterygoid plates and superior constrictor muscle and medial to the zygoma and ascending ramus of the mandible. The pterygoid muscles form its anterior extent and the articular tubercle of the temporal bone, glenoid fossa and styloid process form its posterior limit. It includes the pharyngeal space, i.e. the internal carotid artery, the internal jugular vein, the IXth, Xth and XIth cranial nerves, and the masticator space containing the maxillary branch of the trigeminal nerve, internal maxillary artery, pterygoid venous plexus and pterygoid muscles. The foramina of the skull base, i.e. the carotid canal, jugular foramen, foramen spinosum, foramen ovale, and foramen lacerum, connect it intracranially with the middle fossa. Medially it communicates with the pterygopalatine fossa via the pterygomaxillary fissure, which communicates with the inferior orbital fissure and thus the orbit. It is through these foramina and connections that tumors can spread into and out of the infratemporal fossa.

The infratemporal fossa and associated skull base are invaded by many head and neck cancers as well as being the source of primary malignant tumors in their own right. Such invading cancers include those of the parotid, nasopharynx, temporal bone, paranasal sinus (probably the commonest), skin, and olfactory epithelium as well as metastases from other sites. Intracranial tumors may also grow inferiorly to invade it. Additionally, there are benign tumors that can involve this space, e.g. jugular paragangliomas, meningiomas, and parapharyngeal neuromas.

In cancer surgery, good control of the margins of the tumor is paramount. Traditionally, this is achieved by en bloc excision. This is not always feasible for the skull base, where, as with endoscopic laryngeal surgery, the excision is often achieved in sequential stages with frozen section control where possible.

The essence of skull base surgery is to remove bone rather than retract brain. This allows extensive surgery to be performed while minimizing morbidity. The principle has been extended to endoscopic skull base surgery, including that of the infratemporal fossa. The transnasal endoscopic approaches for malignant tumors are not only useful for palliation but are also advantageous when used in addition to an open approach for tumor resection. However, increasingly the endoscope is being used for complete resection (see also Chapters 12 and 13).

The approaches to the infratemporal fossa and skull base are either lateral or anterior. Superior approaches can be practiced, but they are not usually indicated for benign tumors. They are used as an adjunct to the inferior approach in order to resect involved dura or brain infiltrated by malignant disease.

Surgical approaches are therefore designed not only to remove the tumor but also to identify and preserve crucial vessels and nerves and allow secure closure of any cerebrospinal fluid (CSF) leaks. The reconstruction must be considered at the same time as a decision regarding operability (curative or palliative) and the approach to be employed.

Preoperative assessment

Preoperatively, the cranial nerves must be examined clinically and both CT scan and MRI are always required. Angiography may also be required to image and assess the vascular anatomy and function of the area.

If there is tumor involvement of nerves or vessels the possibility of sacrifice of these and the subsequent rehabilitation of the patient needs to be discussed with the family and patient preoperatively. If the internal carotid artery is considered for sacrifice, which is unusual, then balloon occlusion tests should be undertaken to assess the likely neurological result of such a maneuver. The necessity for sacrifice is usually a contraindication to surgery.

Anterior approaches

Endoscopy, biopsy, and appropriate imaging enable the depth of the tumor, its histological type and the positions of the internal carotid arteries to be defined.

The surgical approaches to the anterior skull base can be divided into open and endoscopic (see Chapters 12 and 13). The open approach used depends on the access that is required and how high in the skull base the tumor is. The anterior skull base, clivus and upper cervical spine are approached from an anterior perspective, the most common operation used being a bifrontal craniotomy. This has the significant advantage that a large pericranial flap can be used to separate the brain from the nasal cavity and this is one of the most reliable flaps that is available. For tumors more inferiorly or posteriorly positioned such as those of the pituitary fossa, base of sphenoid, clivus, or postnasal space the most common open procedure is a maxillary swing operation that allows excellent exposure of these areas.

Many of the tumors that involve this area are malignant and will often require removal of a significant volume of tissue; reconstruction in such cases can only really be achieved with a free flap, bringing in vascularized tissue from elsewhere in the body.

Lateral approach

The lateral approach to the infratemporal fossa again depends on the nature as well as position of the tumor. If a tissue diagnosis is not made preoperatively then frozen sections are required. The extent of the resection will depend upon the type of malignancy; squamous carcinomas and adenocarcinomas requiring a significant resection margin, possibly including the nerves of the foramina of the skull base, while chondrosarcomas need less radical resections.

While the infratemporal fossa can be approached in its entirety using the lateral techniques devised by Fisch, the position of the internal carotid artery relative to the tumor may indicate the need for an anterior approach. In general if the tumor is lateral or posterior to the internal carotid artery, a lateral approach should be used with a preauricular or postauricular incision extending from the neck up to well above the ear. If it is medial to the internal carotid artery consideration should be given to an anterior approach such as maxillary swing or even a mandibulotomy with a lower lip splitting incision. **Figure 17.1** shows a variety of skull approaches.

Endoscopic approach

Endoscopic procedures are increasing in their usage and have the advantages over open surgery of being able to access areas with good visualization, minimal traction and less likely damage to neurovascular structures and the brain. Such endoscopic approaches are not just a different method of visualization, but they require a very different mindset from open or microscopic surgery. There are still some major problems particularly in relation to the control of bleeding. This must always be prepared for the availability of interventional vascular radiology is important.

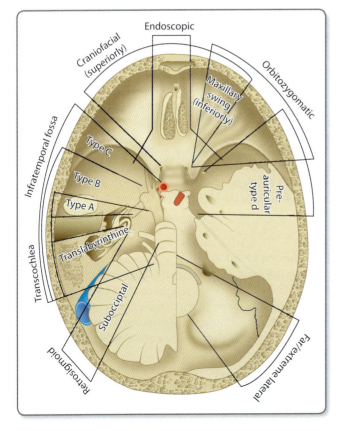

Figure 17.1 Skull base approaches.

The endoscopic approaches (**Figure 17.2**) can be divided into the following:

- The transnasal approaches to the cribriform plate or to the clivus or odontoid peg
- The trans-sphenoidal approaches, i.e. an extension of endoscopic pituitary surgery, accessing the pituitary, the suprasellar cistern, the upper third of the clivus and the area medial to the cavernous sinus
- The transethmoidal approaches through the fovea ethmoidalis, the orbit and the sphenoid to gain access to the anterior fossa, orbital apex and the medial or lateral parts of the cavernous sinus
- The transmaxillary approach is effectively a transpterygoid approach via the pterygopalatine fossa to the infratemporal fossa, Meckel's cave and petrous apex. This approach while described as minimally invasive involves extensive surgery and despite current enthusiasm has yet to be proven safe in many hands

Consent for surgery and operability

Consent for surgery must be realistic, both in terms of the prospects of cure or palliation and with regards to the risks of neural and vascular damage. Care must be taken in managing both the patients' and their

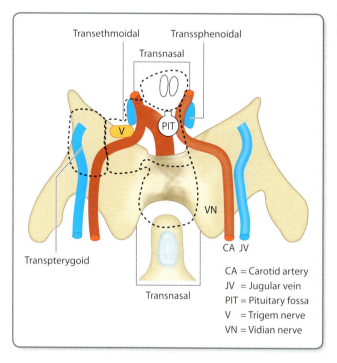

Figure 17.2 Schematic diagram of endoscopic anterior approaches.

relatives' expectations. As to operability, there are case reports of almost every tumor type, no matter how extensive, being cured in individual patients. For instance, temporal bone squamous cell carcinomas are cured in a small number of people even with brain invasion of up to 2 cm. However, because of the paucity of large series it is very difficult to provide the patient with an accurate percentage survival figure: advice is often anecdotal. The patient and their relatives must expect recurrence to occur rather than expect it not to occur if they are going to be managed realistically. In the author's opinion, internal carotid artery involvement of > 180° circumference is a contraindication to surgery.

Operative technique

Posteriorly the postauricular transtemporal approach is usually the most posterior approach but the possibility of using the far lateral (extreme lateral) approach which involves removal of part of the foramen magnum and part of C1 vertebra should also be considered. This allows access to the intracranial cavity and clivus through this space while giving control of the vertebral artery. It is generally not used for malignant tumors with the exception of chondrosarcomas and some chordomas but is used for benign tumors such as meningiomas which need good control of the vertebral artery. Likewise the retrosigmoid approach is not usually applicable to malignant lesions.

The postauricular transtemporal approach

Incision

A question mark shaped incision is employed (**Figure 17.3**). This starts well above the ear 2½ cm anterior to the superior margin of the ear canal, runs posteriorly 3–4 cm behind the ear far enough back to allow control of the sigmoid sinus, curving round under the ear and then is extended down into the neck, preferably in a skin crease. Care is taken not to damage the frontal branch of the facial nerve.

Closure of the external auditory meatus

- Elevate the skin flap anteriorly until the superficial parotid fascia is exposed (**Figure 17.4**)
- Transect the external meatus at the junction of its cartilaginous and bony parts
- Dissect the lateral element, which is now part of the skin flap, free of its cartilage to produce a cuff which is then everted using stay sutures to bring it onto the external side of the skin flap
- Close the meatus using interrupted Dexan to leave a blind ending stump. This will avoid the risk of a subsequent external CSF leak
- If previous surgery, e.g. a meatoplasty, negates such a closure then employs an anteriorly based tragal skin flap sutured onto the skin of the concha (**Figure 17.5**)
- Having closed the meatus, remove all the skin of bony meatus complete with the tympanic membrane to avoid a subsequent implantation cholesteatoma

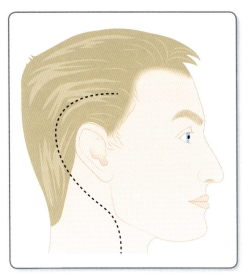

Figure 17.3 Postauricular incision.

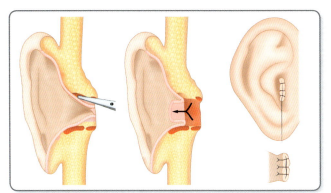

Figure 17.4 Everting a tube of ear canal, skimming and blind sac suturing.

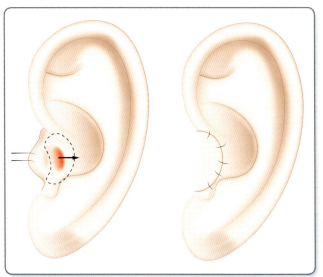

Figure 17.5 Rambo flap using anterior canal wall to suture to conchal bowl for closing ear canal.

Facial nerve exposure

- If oncologically safe to do so, locate the facial nerve at its exit from the stylomastoid foramen as in a standard superficial parotidectomy
- In cases where this would involve entering the tumor field it is advisable to locate one or two branches of the nerve where they leave the gland anteriorly, retracing them retrogradely to the foramen and the main trunk of the nerve
- Having completed a superficial parotidectomy and full exposure of the facial nerve and its branches the zygoma, masseter, and temporalis muscles can be exposed

Neck dissection

- Even if this is not required oncologically, it is necessary for adequate exposure of the major neurovascular structures in the upper neck
- A level 2–4 neck dissection is undertaken with exposure of the internal jugular vein (IJV) and carotid tree (see Chapter 6)
- The posterior belly of the digastric muscle is removed to provide full exposure of the last four cranial nerves, the IJV and the internal carotid artery as they exit the skull base
- The stylohyoid and stylopharyngeus muscles are transacted and the styloid process removed

Bone exposure/mobilization

- The sternomastoid muscle is dissected off the mastoid process (**Figure 17.6**)
- The zygomatic arch is likewise skeletonized
- The temporalis muscle is elevated from its insertion into the skull and reflected anteriorly or inferiorly

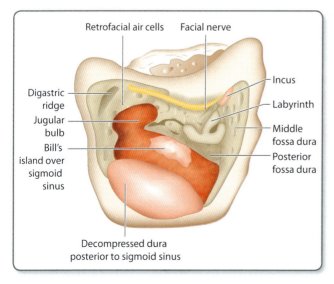

Figure 17.6 Extensive left mastoidectomy.

Retrofacial air cells   Facial nerve

Incus

Digastric ridge

Labyrinth

Jugular bulb

Middle fossa dura

Bill's island over sigmoid sinus

Posterior fossa dura

Decompressed dura posterior to sigmoid sinus

- If the zygoma requires mobilization, this is undertaken after the creation of an anterior V-shaped osteotomy in the arch and sectioning it vertically posteriorly. (The bony cut is either plated or wired at the end of the procedure.)
- A wide cortical mastoidectomy is undertaken with exposure of the sinodural angle, the mastoid antrum and the digastric ridge inferiorly
- The sigmoid sinus veins are best drilled out with care and diathermized
- The transverse sinus should also be skeletonized to allow control of the sigmoid sinus
- The sigmoid sinus is exposed down to the jugular bulb. It can be sacrificed if necessary, although this should only be done if preoperative angiography has confirmed a contralateral sinus
- The bone of the middle cranial fossa floor is also drilled away to expose the superior petrosal sinus.
- The bony labyrinth is exposed and outlined if it is to be preserved

Facial nerve transposition (may not be necessary)
- Remove the ossicles from the middle ear cleft, retaining an intact stapes footplate
- Skeletonize the facial nerve from the geniculate ganglion to the stylomastoid foramen, where it is difficult to separate the nerve out atraumatically. It may be advisable to mobilize the nerve at this point with a cuff or surrounding soft tissue
- Reflect the nerve forward

Labyrinthectomy (may not be necessary)
- Open and then drill away the horizontal and posterior semicircular canals
- The superior semicircular canal is then obliterated
- The vestibule is opened and the internal auditory meatus (IAM) located. It is anterior to the horizontal part of the facial nerve in the middle ear and runs in approximately a straight line with the external meatus
- Initially work around the IAM without opening it to minimize the likelihood of damage to the VIIth and VIIIth nerves and work in a CSF-free field

Obliteration of the sigmoid sinus and jugular fossa dissection
- Remove all remaining bone covering the sigmoid sinus
- Occlude the superior part of the sinus with direct pressure
- Incise the sinus below this point and pack with crushed muscle sutured into the lumen
- Try to avoid tying off sinus as this necessitates incision of the dura and therefore risks a CSF leak
- Divide and tie off the IJV in the upper neck
- The jugular foramen is opened; bleeding from the inferior petrosal sinus requires very light gentle packing as any pressure will damage the adjacent nerves

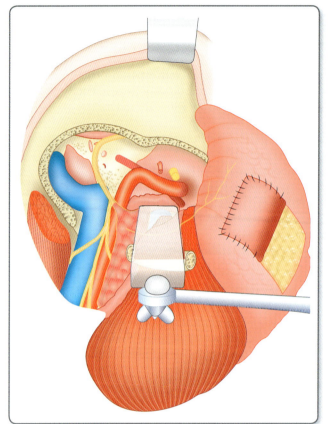

Figure 17.7 Postauricular exposure of the right infratemporal fossa.

Distal control of the ICA

- Remove the basal turn of the cochlea and tensor tympanic muscle (**Figure 17.7**)
- Drill away the bone posterior and superior to the temporomandibular joint
- The mandible can then be mobilized and retracted inferiorly or the condyle removed

Infratemporal fossa dissection

For full access via a type A infratemporal fossa approach anterior translocation of the facial nerve is necessary. For more anterior access (type B and C approaches) further bony work requires the following:

- The temporalis muscle to be elevated inferiorly to expose the infratemporal crest
- Incision of the capsule and removal of the articular disc permits disarticulation of the temporomandibular joint (TMJ)
- Bone of the glenoid fossa and the root of the zygoma are removed completely

- The carotid artery is exposed along its lateral and anterior walls toward the cavernous sinus. Complete exposure allows mobilization out of the carotid canal
- Soft tissue is removed inferiorly from the infratemporal skull base
- Bleeding from the pterygoid plexus is controlled with bipolar diathermy and hemostatic gels
- The pterygoid plates can then be exposed and the infratemporal fossa fully explored

  If access to the nasopharynx and posterior wall of maxillary sinus is needed the pterygoid plates are removed (type C approach).

  Closure and postoperative management:
- Following tumor removal the eustachian tube must be sutured closed to prevent infection from the nasal cavity
- A temporalis muscle flap is used to obliterate the dead space and protect the ICA. Pericranium or a scalp flap may be elevated to protect the infratemporal skull base. Extensive defects are best reconstructed with microvascular free tissue flaps. Mobilized bone is are replaced and fixed in its original position using plates or wire
- Reconstruction of the TMJ is not useful as usually only a minor malocclusion occurs without this whereas very limited mouth opening will occur if reconstruction is attempted

The preauricular infratemporal approach (type D)

- The incision is curved from the temporal area inferiorly in front or behind of the tragus and continues like a parotid incision into the neck (**Figure 17.8**). This has the advantage of being a quick healing incision and avoids any delay in starting postoperative radiotherapy
- Preserve the superficial temporal artery if possible
- The frontal branch of the facial nerve is identified and protected by rolling the superficial layer of the deep temporal fascia with the periosteum over the nerve

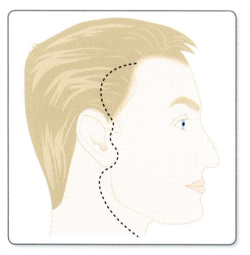

Figure 17.8 Preauricular incision for type D anterior total temporal bone resection.

- The bone of the lateral orbital wall can be removed if required
- The bony work is as detailed above in the postauricular approach with removal of the zygoma, condyle, floor of middle fossa, drilling of the foramen spinosum and foramen ovale and pterygoid plates as required (**Figure 17.9**)
- If the facial nerve is not involved by the tumor, dissection can be undertaken inferiorly as well as superiorly to the nerve, as occurs in a total parotidectomy, but leaving a cuff of tissue around the nerve to minimize traction injury
- If the tumor invades the nerve this dissection is made much easier

Temporal bone cancers

These are treated with surgical resection and postoperative radiotherapy. The resection is either a lateral temporal bone resection or a total temporal bone resection (total petrosectomy).

The extent of these resections is shown in **Figure 17.10** and **Figure 17.11**:

- The lateral temporal bone resection is used for tumors confined to the external ear canal and often involves resection of part of the external ear
- The total temporal bone resection is used for more extensive tumors and those involving the middle ear and mastoid. This resection may need extending into adjacent tissues as dictated by the tumors extent

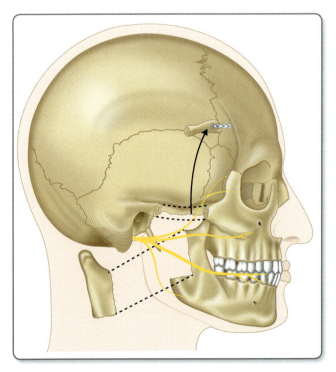

Figure 17.9 Removal of zygoma (to be replaced) and condyle (not to be replaced).

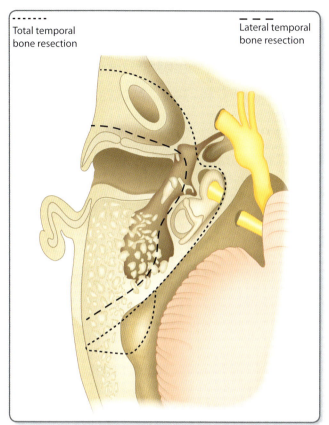

------ Total temporal bone resection

– – – Lateral temporal bone resection

Figure 17.10 Total and lateral temporal bone resection (transverse section).

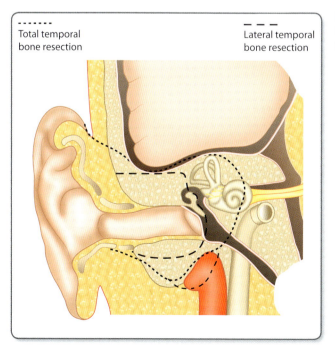

------ Total temporal bone resection

– – – Lateral temporal bone resection

Figure 17.11 Total and lateral temporal bone resection (coronal section).

Surgical procedure

The surgical steps in total temporal bone resection are as follows:
- A postauricular incision isolating the ear canal
- Elevate the skin flaps to completely expose parotid, the zygoma, retromastoid area and neck
- Dissect the facial nerve in a retrograde manner if it is not to be sacrificed
- Perform a neck dissection as required; control the carotid and jugular vessels. Remove soft tissue from mastoid bone
- Reflect masseter from mandible and osteotomize the zygoma and remove the condyle of the mandible
- Reflect temporalis inferiorly
- Divide the styloid muscles
- Undertake a cortical mastoidectomy
- The middle fossa floor is then explored and any involved dura isolated
- Expose the transverse and sigmoid sinuses and, depending on tumor extent, undertake a translabyrinthine or retrosigmoid dissection down to the IAM
- The now isolated temporal bone is detached from the deep attachments using a curved osteotome using two cuts, one superior to inferior toward the IAM and the second from the internal carotid posteriorly, this cut may breach the jugular bulb and some care is needed to gently press on the inferior petrosal sinus to avoid damage to the nerves at the jugular foramen
- When the jugular system is sacrificed the transverse sinus is blocked with crushed muscle sutured into the lumen beforehand
- Hemostasis is secured and residual tumor looked for and removed
- Free flaps to the cavity are required if there is insufficient temporalis or temporoparietal tissue available
- Facial nerve gating, tarsorrhaphy and possible percutaneous endoscopic gastrostomy are employed as required

Complications

Specific complications include CSF leaks, neurological damage, neurovascular damage, wound problems, trismus, and cosmetic deformity. Blood loss during these procedures can be significant.

Apart from neurological deficits, the biggest postoperative problem is the occurrence of a CSF leak. Meticulous closure and reconstruction of the skull base is required to separate the brain from the upper respiratory tract and from the skin. At the end of every operation a gentle Valsalva's maneuver is undertaken to test the closure and/or integrity of the dura. Vascularized tissue is without doubt the best repair. If bone is to be replaced, it can be non-vascularized if under the skin but must have a good blood supply if close to the ear or nose. This is especially true if postoperative radiotherapy is likely to be required. Generally, bony reconstruction is not a good idea unless free vascularized bone grafting is undertaken.

CSF leaks

CSF leaks occur if the dura is violated either intentionally or by tumor invasion. They may also result from hydrocephalus. A watertight dural closure may be difficult to achieve around nerves and vessels, e.g. dura that lies over the cribriform plate can be troublesome because the olfactory nerves travel through it into the nasal cavity. The use of pericranial flaps to repair holes in the dura decreases the risk of CSF leaks. Other vascularized flaps, e.g. temporalis muscle flaps, temporoparietal flaps, radial forearm free flaps, rectus abdominis muscle free flaps, or lateral thigh free flaps are used when appropriate.

Most CSF leaks can be managed non-surgically by placement of a pressure dressing and a spinal drain to diminish the CSF pressure. Surgical exploration and repair of the dural defect may be necessary if the CSF leak does not resolve within a week. Care must be taken to confirm that a pressurized CSF leak is B-transferrin positive before surgical intervention, as it is common for abnormally profuse rhinorrhea or other serous leaks to be misinterpreted as CSF.

Neurological damage

The location of the tumor determines which cranial nerves are at risk. Traction injury, thermal injury due to diathermy or cutting nerves can occur. Cranial nerves displaced by or under tension from tumor growth are most vulnerable, but any cranial nerve in or near the operative field is at risk.

The trigeminal nerve is the most commonly damaged nerve in surgery of the ITF. The loss of corneal sensation, especially in someone with facial nerve dysfunction, greatly increases the risk of a corneal abrasion or exposure keratitis.

Temporary or permanent facial nerve dysfunction is also common after transposition in infra temporal fossa dissection.

Injury to, or sacrifice of, the lower cranial nerves (IX, X, XI, XII) can produce swallowing difficulties and can place the patient at risk for aspiration and pneumonia.

Intraoperatively cranial nerves can be monitored. The facial nerve is frequently monitored using electromyography as are the lower cranial nerves, and the auditory nerve can be monitored with brainstem auditory evoked responses.

Neurovascular damage

Postoperative cerebral ischemia may result from surgical occlusion of the ICA, temporary vasospasm or thromboembolic phenomenon. Surgical dissection of the ICA can injure the vessel wall, resulting in immediate or delayed rupture and hemorrhage from pseudoaneurysm formation. If damage has occurred intraoperatively then consideration should be given to the use of postoperative occlusion or coiling.

Neurological morbidities include the following:

- CSF leak
- Meningitis

- Cerebral contusion and edema
- Pneumocephalus
- Intracranial hemorrhage
- Hydrocephalus
- Cerebral infarction/stroke
- Seizures
- Diabetes insipidus
- Altered mental status
- Anosmia

Wound-related complications

Wound complications include the following:
- Cellulitis
- Infected cranial bone flap or osteomyelitis
- Oronasal fistula
- Necrosis of a pericranial flap
- Encephalocele
- Crusting of the nasal cavity

Chronic sinusitis may result from infection secondary to, loss of sinus mucociliary transport, and obstruction or stenosis of the sinus ostia. In addition, nasal airway stenosis may occur.

Trismus

Trismus occurs commonly due to postoperative pain or to scarring of the pterygoid musculature and TMJ remnant. Trismus improves with regularly performed stretching exercises.

Cosmetic complications

Cosmetic complications include enophthalmos, facial scar, burr hole-related scalp depression, and ocular dystopia. Cosmetic deformity is more likely with anterior surgical approaches because they may involve the orbit or face. After surgery, the position of the eye and the contour of the facial structures should be maintained.

Further reading

Fisch U. The infratemporal fossa approach for the lateral skull base. In: The otolaryngologic Clinics of North America. Philadelphia, PA: WB Saunders Co, 1984:513–52.

Fisch U, Mattox D. Microsurgery of the Skull Base. New York: Thieme Medical Publishers Inc, 1988.

Kassam AB, Gardner P, Snyderman C, Mintz A, Carrau R. Expanded endonasal approach: fully endoscopic, completely transnasal approach to the middle third of the clivus, petrous bone, middle cranial fossa, and infratemporal fossa. Neurosurg Focus 2005; 19:E6.

Mansour OI, Carrau RL, Snyderman CH, Kassam AB. Preauricular infratemporal fossa surgical approach: modifications of the technique and surgical indications. Skull Base 2004; 14:143–51.

R. James A. England

Thyroid cancer is the commonest endocrine neoplasm. It is estimated that there were 44,670 new diagnoses in the United States in 2010 (Altekruse et al. 2010). It is estimated that the lifetime risk of developing thyroid cancer in the United Kingdom is 1 in 243 for women and 1 in 650 for men (Sasieni et al. 2011).

Thyroid cancer is increasing in incidence; in the United Kingdom, age standardized incidence rates have more than doubled from 1.5 to 3.1 per 100,000 persons between 1975–1977 and 2006–2008. Although the reasons for this increase are unclear it is believed that this is partly due to improved pickup and partly due to altered environmental factors.

In autopsy specimens, the incidence of occult thyroid malignancy is much higher, being as high as 35.6% (Harach et al. 1985).

Thyroid cancers are divided into differentiated thyroid cancers, which are those that arise from thyroid follicular cells and retain thyroid differentiation, medullary thyroid cancers (MTCs), which arise from parafollicular C cells, thyroid lymphomas and anaplastic thyroid cancers.

Distant tumors may also metastasize to the thyroid, the commonest being renal cell carcinomas (48.1%), colorectal cancers (10.4%), lung cancers (8.3%) and breast cancers (7.8%) (Chung et al. 2012).

By far the commonest tumor subtype is the differentiated carcinoma that accounts for over 90% of all new diagnoses (Davies et al. 2006).

The etiology of thyroid cancer is unclear, several oncogenes such as RET and TRK rearrangements, BRAF and RAS mutations, and PAX8-PPARγ translocations are important. In addition, there are certain well-recognized risk factors. These include the following:

- *Benign thyroid disease:* Thyroid adenoma, goiter, thyroiditis. One in five thyroid cancers occurs in someone who has had one of these benign conditions
- *Exposure to radiation:* This risk factor is particularly significant in the growing thyroid. It often takes one to two decades to result in

malignant transformation. External beam radiotherapy to the neck in childhood and the Chernobyl disaster both demonstrate this effect. Chernobyl resulted in an explosion in childhood thyroid cancer in the Ukraine

- *Family history:* It is estimated that the risk of developing differentiated thyroid cancer is four to five times greater in a family member of a differentiated thyroid cancer sufferer. In addition, certain genetic mutations increase risk. One such genetic condition is familial adenomatous polyposis
- *Body mass index (BMI):* There is evidence that people with a higher BMI have an increased risk of developing differentiated thyroid cancer
- Acromegaly also leads to an increased risk

Although the overall prognosis for thyroid cancer is extremely good, this is heavily dependent on patient age, tumor subtype, extra thyroidal spread and distant metastases.

The prognostic statistics are somewhat skewed by the ubiquitous low-risk differentiated thyroid cancers that carry an almost universally excellent prognosis. Poorer prognosis tumors are frequently under-treated as a result leading to, in some instances, unnecessary morbidity and mortality.

Differentiated thyroid cancer

Differentiated thyroid cancers are those that arise from the thyroid follicular cell. There are two predominant types, papillary and follicular cancers:

1. Papillary thyroid cancer (PTC) is by far the commonest thyroid cancer accounting for approximately 80% of all thyroid cancers and occurring in 36% of autopsy specimens in one study:
   a. Histopathological features include 'Orphan Annie' nuclei, nuclear grooves and inclusions and Psammoma bodies
   b. PTC is frequently multifocal. There are a number of PTC variants. Some, such as tall cell variant and diffuse sclerosing variant, have a worse prognosis
   c. Tumor metastasis tends to occur via lymphatic spread and metastatic lymphadenopathy is common
2. Follicular thyroid cancer is the second commonest thyroid cancer subtype accounting for approximately 10% of all thyroid cancers:
   a. Metastases tend to be blood borne so distant metastases are more common than in PTC, particularly to bone and lung
   b. The prognosis in differentiated thyroid cancer is generally good. There are many prognostic schemes for risk stratifying patients with carcinomas derived from follicular thyroid cells. However, a recent review suggests that the MACIS system followed by the TNM staging system (**Table 18.1**) are the most accurate predictors of cause specific survival (Lang et al. 2007)

Table 18.1 TNM staging system for thyroid cancer (Edge et al. 2010)	
Tx	Primary tumor cannot be assessed
T0	No evidence of primary tumor
T1a	Tumor ≤ 1 cm in greatest dimension limited to the thyroid
T1b	Tumor > 1 cm but ≤ 2 cm in greatest dimension limited to the thyroid
T2	Tumor > 2 cm but ≤ 4 cm in greatest dimension limited to the thyroid
T3	Tumor > 4 cm in greatest dimension limited to the thyroid or tumor with minimal extrathyroid extension (e.g. extension to sternothyroid muscle or perithyroid soft tissues)
T4a	Tumor of any size extending beyond the thyroid capsule to invade subcutaneous soft tissues, larynx, traches, esophagus, or recurrent laryngeal nerve
T4b	Tumor invades prevertebral fascia or encases carotid artery or mediastinal vessels.
cT4a	Intrathyroidal anaplastic thyroid cancer
cT4b	Anaplastic carcinoma with gross extrathyroid extension
Nx	Regional lymph nodes cannot be assessed
N0	No regional lymph node metastases
N1a	Metastases to level VI
N1b	Metastases to unilateral, contralateral or bilateral cervical (levels I–V) or retropharyngeal or superior mediastinal nodes (level VII)
M0	No distant metastases
M1	Distant metastases

    c. MACIS considers the variables distant metastases, age, completeness of resection, extrathyroid Invasion and primary tumor size. These are used in a weighted equation to calculate a score; the lower the score, the better the prognosis

Presentation

The commonest mode of presentation is a patient with a thyroid swelling:

- Although asymmetrical goiter is common, suspicion should be raised if the patient is under 25 or over 60 years of age, if the patient has a past history of radiation exposure, particularly in early life, and if the patient has a family history of thyroid cancer
- 'Red flag' symptoms include hoarseness, hemoptysis, and stridor

Investigations

The mainstay investigation of the thyroid nodule is fine needle aspiration cytology. This will indicate the nature of the nodule and suggest the extent, if any, of thyroid resection required. Ideally this may be performed under ultrasound control so that the nodule(s) sampled are characterized first.

In addition, patients should undergo a baseline thyroid-stimulating hormone measurement and, in the case of thyroid cancer, a neck ultrasound for nodal involvement.

The necessity of further imaging will be dictated by the presence of retrosternal goiter and nodal metastases, in which case CT of the neck and thorax is recommended, without contrast to avoid the risk of 'stunning' that theoretically reduces the efficacy of postoperative radioactive iodine (**Figure 18.1**).

Treatment

The mainstay of treatment for differentiated thyroid cancer is surgical resection, and completeness of resection has been shown to be an independent prognostic factor (Hay et al. 1993).

Postsurgery, currently most patients receive radioiodine ablation therapy to 'mop up' residual thyroid tissue. However, the role of radioactive iodine ablation (RAI) is controversial on two levels. Firstly, there is no convincing evidence that it adds benefit in the management of low-risk tumors. Secondly, RAI does have side effects, principally sialadenitis, and carries a small long-term carcinogenic risk.

A recent UK-based study, the HiLo trial, has shown that a smaller dose of RAI than previously employed is required to achieve adequate thyroid bed ablation that may lead to reduced treatment-associated morbidity (Mallick et al. 2008).

Medullary thyroid cancer

MTC comprises approximately 3–4% of thyroid cancers.

The cancer arises from parafollicular calcitonin producing C cells that exist predominantly in the middle and upper third of the thyroid gland.

It is a disease with a worse prognosis overall than differentiated thyroid cancer, and as such requires more aggressive surgery.

Approximately, 25% of cases are inherited in which case it is an autosomally dominant disease and can occur as part of multiple endocrine neoplasia (MEN) type 2a (the commonest), MEN 2b or in familial non-MEN MTC. In MEN syndromes, MTC occurs in 100% of patients.

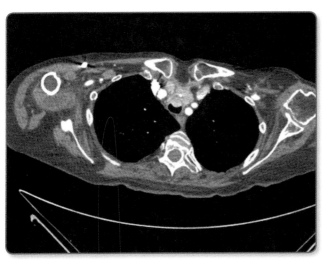

Figure 18.1 Axial CT of mediastinum showing frank tracheal invasion by a PTC, the patients presenting symptom was hemoptysis.

All new MTC diagnoses should be screened for RET proto oncogene mutations to identify/exclude familial disease.

If familial disease has not been excluded, preoperative workup must include screening for other potentially associated neuroendocrine tumors, particularly pheochromocytoma and parathyroid hyperplasia.

A baseline calcitonin and carcinoembryonic antigen (CEA) is also advisable to monitor treatment response and prognosis. Calcitonin is an extremely sensitive tumor marker. Levels of 10–40 pg/mL are suggestive of local nodal involvement. Levels of 150–400 pg/mL suggest distant metastases (Machens et al. 2005).

Once a patient is diagnosed with familial MTC, first-line relatives should undergo genetic testing. If they are found to be gene positive then a prophylactic thyroidectomy is advisable. The age at which this operation will cure the cancer by avoiding its development is dependent on the codon mutation (Machens et al. 2003). Affected individuals who are beyond recommended age should have surgery as soon as possible.

Anaplastic thyroid cancer

Anaplastic thyroid cancer is the most aggressive and rarest of thyroid malignancies. It comprises 1–2% of all thyroid malignancy and tends to occur in patients over 65 years of age.

It is commoner in women than men with a 7:3 split. However, it contributes 14–50% of mortality from thyroid cancer with a 3–5 month median survival rate (Nagaiah et al. 2011).

Presentation is generally with a rapidly expanding neck mass often with associated dysphagia, pain, hoarseness, or stridor. Treatment, depending on degree of local invasion, currently involves surgical resection/debulking where feasible with associated chemoradiotherapy.

Currently doxorubicin is the agent most frequently used with a response rate of 22%; however, trials involving tyrosine kinase inhibitors (TKIs) and antiangiogenic agents are underway.

A Surveillance Epidemiology and End Results (SEER) study suggests that the only prognostic variables are age < 60, intrathyroid tumor and multimodality therapy combining surgery and radiotherapy (Gilliland et al. 1997).

Thyroid lymphoma

Occurring mainly in the sixth decade, thyroid lymphoma is commoner in women and accounts for approximately 5% of thyroid malignancy.

The risk of developing thyroid lymphoma is 70 times higher in patients with Hashimoto's thyroiditis. The majority are non-Hodgkins B-cell lymphomas. Presentation is similar to that of anaplastic thyroid cancer and fine needle aspiration (FNA) may not distinguish the two, leading to the necessity for core or open biopsy. Treatment involves using radiotherapy and/or chemotherapy (Sehn 2005).

Management of thyroid cancer

The mainstay management of nearly all differentiated thyroid cancers (DTCs) is to achieve locoregional control surgically through total thyroidectomy with or without therapeutic lymph node resection.

Most DTCs will receive adjuvant radioiodine ablation to the thyroid bed although certain low-risk tumors may be managed by thyroid lobectomy alone.

Poorer prognosis tumors will require more extensive surgery, involving selective lymph node resection and resection of locally involved structures. These tumors will have a lower incidence of iodine avidity and therefore a higher likelihood of requiring external beam radiotherapy.

MTC is also treated primarily by surgical intervention.

The aim of surgery is to achieve both biochemical and clinical cure hence minimizing recurrence.

In MEN and familial cases, because of the high incidence of lymph node metastases, the most appropriate minimum operation is a total thyroidectomy and bilateral central compartment neck dissection. Such nodal surgery will lead to an increased risk of recurrent laryngeal nerve damage and hypoparathyroidism. In such cases, parathyroid autotransplantation should be considered if the blood supply to the inferior parathyroids is impaired.

Lateral nodal surgery (levels 2a–5b) will be necessary in image positive disease and when stimulated calcitonin levels dictate (**Figure 18.2**).

Surgery for anaplastic thyroid cancer will rarely result in macroscopic clearance.

However, debulking the tumor burden is the therapeutic mainstay, followed by adjuvant therapy in an attempt to reduce morbidity and prolong survival. The prognosis, however, still remains dismal.

Surgery for thyroid cancer

Thyroid lobectomy

The patient is sat up preoperatively in the neutral position and the neck marked for incision level. This is at the bony soft tissue junction at the sternal notch. The symmetrical incision is extended horizontally cutting the medial upper border of the clavicle on each side (**Figure 18.3**).

With the patient supine with 30° of reverse Trendelenberg, neck extension should be achieved with the use, where possible, of a head ring and sandbag.

An incision is made through skin and platysma. In most instances, this need only be 5 cm in length.

A superior subplatysmal flap is raised by forcing a 6 × 4 gauze swab under platysma and upward along the surface of both sternomastoid muscles. The central part of the flap is then raised in the same way. This results in a rapid and bloodless dissection.

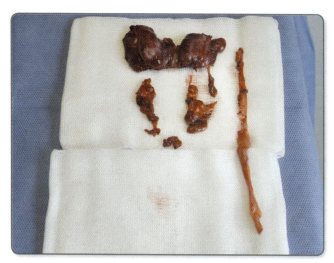

Figure 18.2 Minimum operation in MEN 2a MTC; total thyroidectomy, bilateral level 6–7 nodal clearance (bilateral thymic remnants have also been removed and are on the right). An enlarged right inferior parathyroid is also seen (removed to treat associated parathyroid hyperplasia).

The linea alba is divided from the sternal notch to approximately 1 cm above the cricoid cartilage.

Blunt dissection is performed to free the thyroid lobe from below the strap muscles. This is best achieved by pulling the lobe medially up and onto the trachea with a gauze covered finger while simultaneously getting an assistant to retract the straps laterally with a Langenbeck retractor.

The middle thyroid vein can normally be separated from the lobe with diathermy.

The superior thyroid pole is then separated from the cricothyroid muscle. This is done by retracting the pole laterally to open Jolls' triangle.

The vessels forming the superior vascular pedicle are then divided individually as the superior pole is dissected free. This may be done with bipolar diathermy in most cases although vessels of 5 mm or greater may need a liga clip.

Care must be taken to dissect with the pole retracted laterally (this is best achieved using a Babcock retractor) to minimize risk of injury to the external branch of the superior laryngeal nerve, which supplies the cricothyroid muscle.

Once the superior pole is dissected down to the level of the cricoid cartilage (the dissection must not go below as this may endanger the recurrent laryngeal nerve), the lobe may be rolled up and onto the trachea.

As the lobe is gently retracted medially with a Langenbeck retractor retracting the ipsilateral strap muscles and carotid sheath laterally, fibrous bands causing adherence of the lobe to the strap muscles and carotid sheath are divided by tension and opening the dissecting scissors in a parallel plane to the bands at 90° to the midline. Bands that do not divide in this way are generally vessels under tension and these may be diathermized.

Once the posterior extent of the lobe is identified, a silk stay suture is placed through the lobe in a cephalocaudal orientation, this is retracted

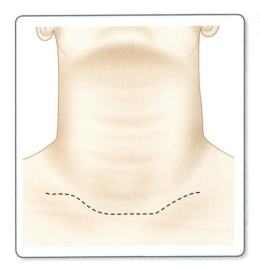

Figure 18.3 Surgical thyroidectomy incision (dashed line) at the bony soft tissue junction.

medially by an assistant. The search for the recurrent laryngeal nerve and the parathyroid glands may now proceed.

The right recurrent laryngeal nerve runs approximately 45° inferolaterally from the cricoid. On the left side, it has a more vertical relationship. The dissection is layer by layer and achieved with the use of Metzenbaum scissors and Adsons' toothed forceps.

Once identified, the superior parathyroid is normally seen on or just above the nerve at the level of the cricoid. Dissection proceeds superficial to the nerve and medial to the parathyroid to minimize the risk of devascularization of the parathyroid.

The lobe is dissected free from the trachea caudally and no search is made for the inferior parathyroid, as this risks devascularization. However, the inferior pole of the lobe is carefully inspected to ensure the inferior gland is not being inadvertently removed.

If an inferior gland is seen on the inferior pole, this is dissected off using bipolar diathermy and care is taken to maintain a soft tissue pedicle.

The posterior suspensory ligament of the thyroid (Berry's ligament) is then diathermized and cut with a 15 blade to deliver the thyroid lobe.

The inferior thyroid artery is never ligated/divided laterally, as this will devascularize the parathyroids. Devascularization of the thyroid is performed in a subcapsular manner wherever possible medial to the parathyroids.

Level 6–7 dissection

It is important to first establish whether a level 6–7 dissection is necessary. In low-risk disease it seldom is, and performing this surgery will increase the risk of recurrent laryngeal nerve (RLN) injury and permanent hypoparathyroidism.

It is best to perform this procedure after thyroidectomy, when the RLN is exposed near to the cricoid.

To begin, all fibrofatty tissue superficial to the RLN is removed from trachea medially to carotid laterally.

The dissection should include all lymphoid tissue from the hyoid down, removing all fibrofatty tissue from the laryngeal skeleton, and ensuring any thyroglossal tract remnants are removed.

The inferior extent of the dissection is unclear. There is no physiological boundary between levels 6 and 7; so when central nodal clearance is necessary, both areas should be cleared.

Realistically this involves following the common carotid arteries as far behind the manubrium as is possible without performing a sternotomy, down to the brachiocephalic trunk on the right and toward the aorta on the left.

In high-risk patients, when preoperative imaging confirms mediastinal nodal disease, sternotomy is necessary to adequately clear the area. This is more pertinent in MTC.

Adjuvant therapy

The mainstay adjuvant therapy for DTC is radioiodine (RAI) ablation. Firstly, this is used to destroy any remaining normal thyroid tissue increasing the sensitivity of further RAI imaging and the specificity of thyroglobulin measurements. Secondly, it destroys any microscopic carcinoma and improves outcome, permitting postablation scanning to identify any remaining areas of residual malignancy. It is given 4–6 week postsurgery.

In higher risk cancers, dedifferentiation may have occurred and RAI avidity is reduced. In this scenario, external beam radiotherapy may be necessary although the survival benefit it confers is unclear.

External beam radiotherapy is also used in MTC and anaplastic thyroid cancer, although the therapeutic benefits are limited.

When all other options have failed and disease is progressive in DTC, chemotherapeutic agents are used, doxorubicin being the commonest. TKIs such as sorafenib are therapeutic modalities that have recently become available.

In MTC, somatostatin analogue therapy is used for symptom control. The TKI vandetanib is approved by the FDA in metastatic and locally unresectable MTC.

Follow-up

Follow-up of thyroid cancer involves clinical assessment with regular thyroglobulin monitoring for DTC and calcitonin and CEA monitoring for MTC. Due to the risk of late recurrence, follow-up is normally lifelong.

In DTC, thyroxine replacement is deliberately supraphysiological (TSH 0.1–0.5 mU/L) until apparent remission is achieved in low-risk patients, and TSH suppression is maximized (TSH <0.1 mU/L) for 3–5 years in high-risk patients (Pacini et al. 2006). This is to reduce the pituitary 'drive' on any residual thyroid tissue.

References

Altekruse S, Kosary C, Krapcho M, et al. SEER Cancer Statistics Review, 1975–2007. Bethesda, MD: National Cancer Institute, 2010.

Chung AY, Tran TB, Brumund KT, et al. Metastases to the thyroid: a review of the literature from the last decade. Thyroid 2012; 22:258–68.

Davies L, Welch HG. Increasing incidence of thyroid cancer in the United States, 1973–2002. J Am Med Assoc 2006; 295:2164–7.

Edge SB, Byrd DR, Compton, et al. AJCC cancer staging manual, 7th edn. New York, NY: Springer, 2010:87–96.

Gilliland FD, Hunt WC, Morris DM, Key CR. Prognostic factors for thyroid carcinoma: a population-based study of 15,698 cases from the Surveillance, Epidemiology and End Results (SEER) program 1973–1991. Cancer 1997; 79:564–73.

Harach HR, Franssila KO, Wasenius VM. Occult primary carcinoma of the thyroid: a 'normal' finding in Finland. Cancer 1985; 56:531–8.

Hay ID, Bergstralh EJ, Goellner JR, et al. Predicting outcome in papillary thyroid carcinoma: development of a reliable prognostic scoring system in a cohort of 1779 patients surgically treated at one institution during 1940 through 1989. Surgery 1993; 114:1050–57.

Lang BH, Lo CY, Chan WF, et al. Staging systems for papillary thyroid carcinoma: a review and comparison. Ann Surg 2007; 245:366–78.

Machens A, Schneyer U, Holzhausen HJ, Dralle H. Prospects of remission in medullary thyroid carcinoma according to basal calcitonin level. J Clin Endocrinol Metab 2005; 90:2029–34.

Mallick U, Harmer C, Hackshaw A. The HiLo Trial: a multicentre randomised trial on high- versus low-dose radioiodine, with or without recombinant human thyroid stimulating hormone, for remnant ablation after surgery for differentiated thyroid cancer. Clin Oncol 2008; 20:325–26.

Nagaiah G, Hossain A, Mooney CJ, et al. Anaplastic thyroid cancer: a review of epidemiology, pathogenesis and treatment. J Oncol 2011; 2011:542358.

Sasieni PD, Shelton J, Ormiston-Smith N, et al. What is the lifetime risk of developing cancer?: The effect of adjusting for multiple primaries. Br J Cancer 2011; 105:460–65.

Sehn LH, Donaldson J, Chhanabhai M, et al. Introduction of combined CHOP plus rituximab therapy dramatically improved outcome of diffuse large B cell lymphoma in British Columbia. J Clin Oncol 2005; 23:5027–33.

Paolo Matteucci

Skin cancer is the most common form of cancer and accounts for approximately a third of all cancers. It is broadly divided into melanoma skin cancer (MSC) and non-melanoma skin cancer (NMSC). The majority of skin cancers that present on the head and neck are NMSCs and 75% of these are basal cell carcinomas (BCC). Squamous cell carcinoma makes up the majority of the remaining tumors, followed by melanoma and a variety of much rarer tumors. As with all cancers cutaneous malignancies should be treated by specialist clinicians and a good prognosis depends on appropriate timely care.

Non-melanoma skin cancer

This includes a wide range of tumors the majority of which are of epithelial origin. The main etiological factor is ultraviolet (UV) light exposure particularly at wavelengths 290–320 nm. The UV radiation causes DNA damage and is particularly potent in those with fair skin whose burn easily and rarely tan. The most common source of this radiation is the sun but prolonged sun-bed use is also a risk factor. Immunosuppression, in particular in those with organ transplants, is also a risk factor, as is previous radiotherapy (see **Table 19.1** for a comprehensive list). Genetic predisposition in terms of a strong family history or conditions such as Gorlin's syndrome or xeroderma pigmentosa also increases the risk.

Diagnosis and staging

The diagnosis of many skin cancers may be clinical but the gold standard is biopsy and histological analysis. In many cases, diagnosis and treatment will be one in the same with a therapeutic excision biopsy. Initial clinical examination must include an examination of the regional lymphatic basins. Staging for all NMSCs is the same and uses the tumor, node and metastasis (TNM) format favored by the American Joint Committee on Cancer (AJCC). Routine radiological assessment is not necessary in the majority of NMSC.

Stage	TNM	Characteristics
Table 19.1 The AJCC staging for SCC and BCC		
Stage 0	Tis N0 M0	The cancer involves only the epidermis and has not spread to the dermis. Squamous cell carcinoma in situ is also called Bowen's disease
Stage I	T1 N0 M0	The cancer is no >2 cm (between $3/4^2$ and $7/8^2$). It has not invaded into muscle, cartilage or bone and has not spread to lymph nodes or other organs
Stage II	T2 T3 N0 or N0 M0 M0	The cancer is >2 cm and has not invaded into muscle, cartilage, or bone and has not spread to lymph nodes or other organs
Stage III	T4 any T N0 or N1 M0 M0	The cancer has grown into tissues beneath the skin (such as muscle, bone, or cartilage) and/or it has spread to regional (nearby) lymph nodes. In this stage, the cancer has not spread to other organs such as the lungs or brain
Stage IV	Any T Any N M1	The cancer can be any size and may or may not have spread to local lymph nodes. It has spread to other organs, such as the lungs or brain

BCC, basal cell carcinomas; SCC, squamous cell carcinomas.

Basal cell carcinoma

This is by far the most common skin cancer. It usually follows a slow, indolent course and is to all intents and purposes a local disease. There are rare reports of metastatic BCC but this occurs in <1 in 1000 cases. However neglected BCCs, particularly in the head and neck are destructive and can be relentless in the local invasion and may present very difficult management challenges. While many BCCs have the classic nodular-cystic appearance with surface telangiectasia, there are a number of subtypes of the tumor that may present diagnostic challenges. The treatment of BCCs broadly falls into surgical and non-surgical.

Destructive surgical treatments

Curettage and cautery

This treatment method is quick, cheap and simple and relies on the heat from cautery destroying residual tumor cells after removal of the main part of the lesion with a sharp curette or blade. It can be effective for small lesions but its use is limited in the head and neck, as it causes unpredictable scarring and is to be avoided in high-risk areas. The main disadvantage of the technique is that no specimen is produced for histological analysis to assess adequacy of margins.

Cryotherapy

Cryotherapy involves the use of liquid nitrogen to destroy tumors. It has similar indications to curettage and cautery and can also result in problematic scarring. It may result in painful blistering swelling. When used in appropriate lesions it can be an effective treatment but once again does not produce a specimen for histological analysis.

Excisional surgical treatments

Simple excision

The mainstay of treatment for BCCs is surgical excision. For tumors <2 cm in size with a discrete border a 3 mm margin is adequate, particularly when marked under magnification and performed by a specialist surgeon. If there is doubt about the borders of the lesion then a 4–5 mm is necessary and will result in a 95% complete excision rate. For lesions >2 cm in diameter, wider margins are required, in some cases up to 15 mm to achieve a 95% complete excision rate. The management of incompletely excised BCCs will depend on the margin involved, how high risk the lesion is and patient preference. In essence low-risk BCCs incompletely excised at a lateral margin may be suitable for observation. If, on the other hand, the lesion is high risk or the deep margin is involved, it is prudent to consider wider excision as the recurrence rate is high and recurrence may be difficult to treat (Telfer et al. 1999). Retreatment may involve further surgery or radiotherapy. In functional sensitive areas such as the perioccular area and eyelids and in particular where complex reconstructions are required frozen section can be used to confirm completeness of excision. Alternatively Mohs' surgery is a highly effective treatment.

Mohs' micrographic surgery

This is a sophisticated technique which has cure rates for BCC of 94–99% at 5 years (Rowe et al. 1989). It is performed by highly trained Mohs' surgeons. The specimen is horizontally sectioned and mapped. If there is residual tumor the involved margin re-excised and the process repeated until there is no residual tumor. In this way, the removal of the tumor is optimized while preserving as much tissue as possible. The disadvantages of Mohs' surgery are that it is time consuming, requires specialized equipment, is expensive and not universally available.

Non-surgical treatments

Radiotherapy

Radiotherapy is a highly effective treatment for BCCs, particularly those of <2 cm diameter. Treatment is time consuming, costly and may be associated with significant morbidity for the patient. However, it may result in better aesthetic and functional outcomes in some areas. It is also of use in lesions treated surgically that have been excised with a narrow or involved margin or are high risk.

Topical treatments

Superficial BCCs may be treated with 5-fluorouracil ointment. In well-selected patients with superficial BCCs cure rates of up to 95% may be achieved. Imiquimod is an immune modulator that upregulates the expression of interferon and can be used topically for superficial BCCs. Both topical treatments can cause florid cutaneous reactions.

Photodynamic therapy

Photodynamic therapy has been used with some success in BCC with clearance rates reported between 82% and 92%. It involves the topical or intratumoral administration of a photosensitizing agent that causes tissue destruction when exposed to light of a particular wavelength. The main drawback is persistent photosensitivity which may last 4–6 weeks.

Squamous cell carcinoma

Squamous cell carcinoma (SCC) is the second most common skin cancer and is commonly found on the head and neck. It has the potential to metastasize. The metastatic potential is higher in patients with tumors on the ear and lip and conversely in tumors developing on areas not exposed to the sun such as the perineum or the sole of the foot. Tumors > 2 cm in diameter or 4 mm in thickness have a higher metastatic potential. Poorly differentiated tumors are also higher risk. Metastatic rates vary from 5% to 50% depending on how high risk the tumor is (Motley et al. 2003). In the majority of cases, the tumors spread to the draining lymph node basin.

Actinic keratoses and Bowen's disease are precursors to SCC. These precursor lesions can be excised or treated with topical therapies such as cryotherapy, 5-fluorouracil and diclofenac ointment with very good effect.

The mainstay of treatment for SCCs is surgical excision. For lesions of 2 cm diameter or less margins of 4–5 mm will result in a 95% complete excision rate. However for larger tumors margins of > 1 cm may be required. Mohs' surgery may be of value.

In the majority of cases a good clinical history and examination will suffice but in large or fixed lesions or where there is a concern about involvement of underlying structure preoperative imaging is advisable.

SCCs on the auricle and external auditory meatus are of particular concern. If they extend into the external auditory canal they can spread down preformed and vascular structures and extend into the middle ear and petrous temporal bone. The aim of treatment is to achieve clear surgical margins but radiotherapy should also be considered. Surgical treatment may involve petrosectomy with sacrifice of the facial nerve and flap reconstruction. Preoperative imaging is essential.

Other non-melanoma skin cancer

A number of much rarer skin tumors can occur. Of these Merkel cell tumors, sebaceous carcinoma, dermatofibrosarcoma protuberans and adnexal carcinomas are the most important. While generally very rare, sebaceous carcinoma is the third most common skin cancer on the eyelid. They can be locally aggressive and metastasize. Wide excision with clear margins and close follow-up are essential. Merkel cell tumors are neuroendocrine tumors that are locally and regionally aggressive. Sentinel node biopsy should be considered. Dermatofibrosarcoma protuberans is a locally aggressive cutaneous sarcoma. Treatment requires wide surgical margins as local recurrence rates are high. Adnexal carcinomas are very rare. Excision with clear margins is the mainstay of treatment with close follow-up.

Staging of SCCs and BCCs

SCCs and BCCs are staged using the tumor (T) node (N) metastasis (M) format.

Primary tumor (T)

- Tx: It is not possible to assess the primary tumor
- T0: There is no evidence of a primary tumor
- Tis: In situ disease
- T1: The tumor is 2 cm or less in maximum diameter.
- T2: The tumor is >2 cm but <5 cm in maximum diameter
- T3: The tumor is >5 cm in maximum diameter
- T4: The tumor invades deeper structures

Nodes (N)

- Nx: The nodes cannot be assessed
- N0: No nodal disease is present
- N1: Nodal disease is present

Metastasis (M)

- Mx: Metastasis cannot be assessed
- M0: No metastasis
- M1: Metastasis

The staging system (**Table 19.1**) is not universally used as it does not take account of the risk factors such as depth of tumor, site or degree of differentiation and so is not an accurate prognostic tool.

Malignant melanoma

Melanoma accounts for only 5% of cutaneous malignancies but 75% of the mortality. Overall, the incidence of melanoma is increasing at about 4–6% per annum. Despite melanoma having an apparently high mortality overall survival is 80% for men and 90% for women in the United Kingdom. About 30% of all melanoma occurs on the head and neck and overall has a poorer prognosis than malignant melanoma (MM) elsewhere on the body. As with other skin cancers MM of the head and neck brings some particular surgical challenges in terms of resection and reconstruction. Between 1% and 3% of melanomas are mucosal and these carry a very poor prognosis. They may occur within the oral cavity, sinonasal tract or within the pharynx. Ocular melanomas also occur very rarely but are outside the scope of this discussion.

Etiology and risk factors

As with other skin cancers exposure to ultraviolet light is a major etiological factor. In particular high intensity intermittent exposure and blistering sunburn before the age of 10 is an independent risk factor. Patients with fair, freckly skin that burns easily are at higher risk as are those with a family history of one or more first degree relatives with melanoma. Patients with large numbers of normal or dysplastic moles have an increased risk although most melanomas do not arise in pre-existing moles. Giant congenital nevus (20 cm in diameter or >2% of body surface area) is associated with an increased risk of developing a MM, but the degree of risk is extremely difficult to assess. A personal history of melanoma increases risk, as does xeroderma pigmentosa.

Diagnosis

Many patients will seek a consultation because a mole has changed or a new pigmented lesion has developed. The American Cancer Service has developed a relatively simple assessment tool which is A: Asymmetry, B: Border, C: Color alteration, D: Diameter >6 mm, E: evolution overtime. Dermoscopy is increasingly being used in clinical practice but definitive diagnosis can only be achieved with biopsy. In general a narrow margin excision biopsy should be employed to allow histological assessment of the entire lesion. One of the most important staging criteria for melanoma is the Breslow thickness and incision biopsy may under stage a tumor by not including the thickest part. The exceptions to this are large Lentigo Malignas where complete excision would cause reconstructive or cosmetic challenges, lesions on the nail beds which require incision biopsy and suspect areas within giant congenital nevi. Histological analysis should include assessment of ulceration, growth phase, Breslow thickness (BT) (measured from granular layer of the epidermis to deepest part of tumor), regression, mitotic count, tumor infiltrating lymphocytes, histological subtype, lymphatic or vascular invasion, margins of excision, perineural invasion, and the presence of microsatellites.

Of these Breslow thickness, mitotic count (for tumors <1 mm thick), ulceration, vascular or perineural invasion and the presence of microsatellites have prognostic value.

Staging

The AJCC system of staging using the TNM system is an accurate prognostic tool.

Primary tumor

- Tx: It is not possible to assess the primary tumor
- T0: There is no evidence of a primary tumor
- Tis: In situ disease
- T1a: BT <1 mm, no ulceration, no mitoses
- T1b: BT <1 mm, with ulceration or mitoses >1 mm^{-2}
- T2a: BT >1 mm <2 mm, no ulceration
- T2b: BT >1 mm <2 mm, with ulceration
- T3a: BT >2 mm <4 mm, no ulceration
- T3b: BT >2 mm <4 mm, with ulceration
- T4a: BT >4 mm no ulceration
- T4b: BT >4 mm with ulceration

Nodes

- Nx: Nodal metastases cannot be assessed
- N0: No nodal metastases

- N1a: 1 node with micrometastasis
- N1b: 1 node with macrometastasis
- N2a: 2–3 nodes with micrometastasis
- N2b: 2–3 nodes with macrometastasis
- N2c: intransit or satellite metastasis without metastatic lymph nodes
- N3: 4 or more nodes or matted nodes or in transit metastasis or satellites with metastatic nodes

Metastasis

- M0: No metastases
- M1a: Distant skin, subcutaneous or lymph node metastases
- M1b: Lung metastases
- M1c: Other visceral metastases or distant metastases with a raised serum lactate dehydrogenase (LDH).
- Advancing stage correlates with poorer prognosis (**Table 19.2**).

Sentinel lymph node biopsy

This has become an integral part of the management of MM. It is a staging tool to identify micrometastatic or occult lymph node involvement. There is no evidence that its use improves survival (Morton et al. 2006). The presence or absence of a metastasis on sentinel lymph node biopsy (SLNB) is a powerful prognostic factor in staging MM. The technique consists of identifying the first draining nodes of the tumor using lymphoscintography preoperatively and an injection of blue dye and the use of a handheld radiation detector to identify the node at the time of the wide excision of the melanoma. It is technically challenging in the neck and may have a higher false

Table 19.2 The AJCC stage for malignant melanoma					
Stage	T	N	M	5-year survival (%)	10-year survival (%)
0	Tx	N0	M0		
IA	T1a	N0	M0	95	87–89
IB	T1b or T2a	N0	M0	88–92	78–85
IIA	T2b or T3a	N0	M0	77–79	62–66
IIB	T3b or T4a	N0	M0	61–70	49–57
IIC	T4b	N0	M0	43–47	31–34
IIIA	T1–T4a	N1a or N2a	M0	57–73	50–67
IIIB	T1–T4b T1–T4a	N1a or N2a N1b, N2b, or N2c	M0	41–57	29–53
IIIC	T1–T4b Any T	N1b, N2b, or N3 N3	M0	20–34	11–29
IV	Any T	Any N	M1	5–22	

AJCC, American Joint Committee on Cancer; TNM, tumor, node and metastasis.

negative rate than other sites. Controversy still exists as to its role and in particular ultrasound assessment and follow-up may prove as effective.

Other staging investigations

For patients with stage III and IV disease, CT staging of the head, thorax, abdomen, and pelvis should be undertaken. For those with stage IV disease the serum LHD should be measured.

Treatment

Wide local excision

The risk of local recurrence is reduced by wide excision, as has been widely demonstrated in the literature. For tumors with a BT < 1 mm a 1 cm margin wider excision should be performed. For whose with a BT between 1 and 2 mm a 2 cm margin, with a BT between 2 and 4 mm a 2–3 cm margin and those thicker than 4 mm a 3 cm margin. There are no studies comparing a 2 and 3 cm margin for tumors thicker than 4 mm and in practice a smaller margin may be taken depending on local factors. Wide excisions in the head and neck will often necessitate complex reconstructions and this must be considered when planning treatment (Marsden 2010).

Neck dissection

There is no place for elective node dissection in the clinically N0 neck. Patients with stage 1b and above may be offered a SLNB as a staging procedure. For patients with positive SLNBs a comprehensive neck dissection should be considered as this may improve local control. In patients with suspicious nodes, fine needle aspiration cytology (FNAC) should be performed, under imaging guidance where appropriate. If this is equivocal and the index of suspicion is high then open biopsy of the node may be appropriate. Comprehensive neck dissection should be performed for all confirmed neck node involvement and for lesions on the face and anterior scalp serious consideration should be made regarding superficial parotidectomy.

Adjuvant treatment

There is good evidence that radiotherapy can improve local control of MM in the head and neck. There is no evidence to suggest it improves survival. A number of therapeutic agents are available for the treatment of stage IV MM. Interferon and ipilimumab are immune modulators that are used in the treatment of advanced melanoma. BRAF inhibitors are very effective in patients with the BRAF gene mutation and stage IV disease and there are trials investigating combination therapies. While these therapies may delay or control recurrence they do not cure the disease.

Summary

Both melanoma and NMSC of the head and neck can present complex diagnostic and therapeutic challenges. These patients are best managed by specialist teams to optimize outcomes.

References

Marsden JR, Newton-Bishop JA, Burrows L, et al. Revised UK guidelines for the management of cutaneous melanoma 2010. J Plast Reconstr Aesthet Surg 2010; 63:1401–19.

Morton DL, Thompson JF, Cochran AJ, et al. Sentinel-node biopsy or nodal observation in melanoma. N Engl J Med 2006; 355:1307–17.

Motley R, Kersey P, Lawrence C. Multiprofessional guidelines for the management of the patient with primary cutaneous squamous cell carcinoma. Br J Plast Surg 2003; 56:85–91.

Rowe DE, Carroll RJ, Day CL Jr. Long-term recurrence rates in previously untreated (primary) basal cell carcinoma: implications for patient follow-up. J Dermatol Surg Oncol 1989; 15:315–28.

Telfer NR, Colver GB, Bowers PW. 1999. Guidelines for the management of basal cell carcinoma. British Association of Dermatologists. Br J Dermatol 1999; 141:415–23.

Surgical reconstruction in the head and neck

Paolo Matteucci

Surgical ablation of malignant tumors of the head and neck may leave large defects that would cause severe functional, psychosocial and aesthetic problems if not reconstructed. In many cases, the options for complex reliable reconstructions have expanded the range of what is considered surgically resectable. The underlying philosophy of reconstructive surgery is to restore function and form, with function carrying the greater importance.

The principles of reconstructive surgery are similar whatever the defect to be rebuilt and are a good place to start the discussion. The first step is assessment. Both the patient and the expected defect need to be assessed. This requires close collaboration between the ablative and reconstructive surgeons, the anesthetist, radiologist, and pathologists as well as in many cases reconstructive dentist, oncologist, speech and language teams, and nutritionists. The patient must be counseled about the surgical options and understand the scale of the surgery and postoperative recovery and also the functional limitations of what may be achieved.

Having established that the patient is suitable for surgery, the planning process is paramount. By reviewing preoperative imaging and pathology, the likely defect that will result from surgery can be estimated and the reconstructive options planned. However, it is not uncommon for intraoperative findings to differ substantially from those expected and flexibility must be part of the preoperative plan.

The questions the reconstructive surgeon must consider are as follow:

1. What will be missing?
2. What functional implication will this have?
3. What must be reconstructed?

4. What reconstructive options are there?
5. What can the patient tolerate?

The reconstructive ladder

The reconstructive ladder is a framework used to assist in selection of reconstructive technique. At the bottom of the ladder are the simplest options such as healing by secondary intention and direct closure and at the top the most complex composite tissue free flaps. Often it is self-apparent which option is correct. For other cases, different options have to be weighed up and more than one technique employed in the same patient (**Table 20.1**).

Skin and soft tissue defects

Small skin and soft tissue defects may be closed directly or may require the use of skin grafts or local flaps (**Figures 20.1–20.6**). Functional and aesthetic outcomes are usually good. Larger defects may require regional, pedicled or free flaps. Anterior and lateral defects may be reconstructed with pectoralis major and deltopectoral flaps (**Figure 20.7**). The lateral and posterior defects may be closed using pedicled latissimus dorsi and trapezius flaps **Figure 20.8**) For larger

Table 20.1 The reconstructive ladder		
Technique	Advantages	Disadvantages
Healing by secondary intention	Simple	Slow, poor scarring, contractures, requires vascularized tissue
Direct closure	Simple, rapid healing may give excellent results	May cause functional or aesthetic deformities Requires sufficient local tissue laxity
Skin graft	Rapid healing, relatively simple May give good aesthetic results	Require well vascularized bed May give poor aesthetic and functional results May have painful donor site
Dermal regeneration templates	May be used in conjunction with split skin grafts on poor recipient sites or to improve functional or aesthetic outcomes	Expensive Expertise required in case selection
Local flap	Rapid healing Good aesthetic results possible	Requires sufficient adjacent tissue or may need a skin graft on the secondary defect More extensive scarring
Regional flap	Relatively straight forward, reliable pedicle, allow surgery to be localized at one body site	Limitations in pedicle length, limitations in tissue type available, poor functional out comes at recipient and donor site
Free flap	Reconstruction tailored to defect Composite tissue transfer Donor morbidity may be minimized Flexibility in placement Simultaneous resection and flap elevation	Technically demanding Time consuming Require adequate recipient vessels Intensive postoperative monitoring Donor site morbidity
Tissue expansion	Can be used with other techniques in the ladder to improve outcome, generates new skin through distraction histiogenesis, excellent aesthetic outcomes	Requires a number of weeks to expand tissue Expanders may extrude and become infected Rarely useful in immediate cancer reconstruction but may be used during revisional surgery

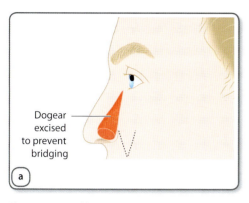 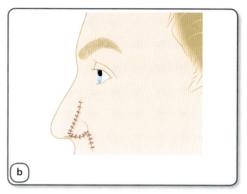

Dogear excised to prevent bridging

Figure 20.1a and b Superiorly based nasolabial flap for a skin tumor of the nasal ala.

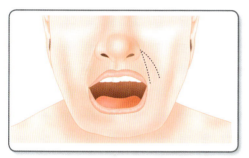 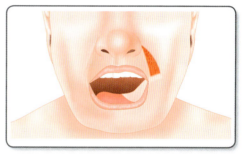

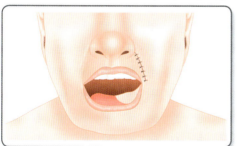

Figure 20.2 Inferiorly based nasolabial flap for a small anterior floor of mouth carcinoma.

Figure 20.3 A wedge excision of an annular tumor, with direct closure.

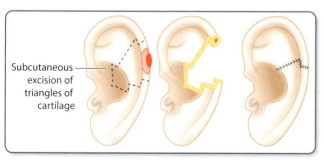

Subcutaneous excision of triangles of cartilage

defects, or those extending superiorly beyond the arc of rotation of pedicled flaps, a free flap may be required; options include the radial forearm flap, anterolateral thigh flap and rectus abdominis

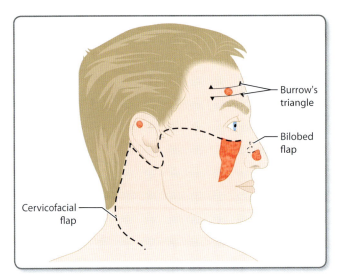

Figure 20.4 A cervicofacial flap, a bilobed flap for a nasal skin tumor and advancement flaps for a tumor of the forehead.

Burrow's triangle

Bilobed flap

Cervicofacial flap

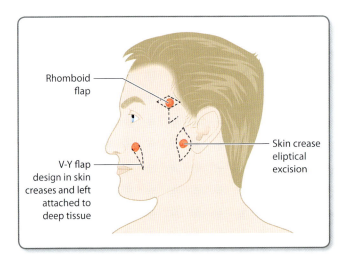

Figure 20.5 A V-Y advancement flap, an elliptical excision of a cheek lesion and a rhomboid flap for a tumor of the skin of the temple.

Rhomboid flap

Skin crease eliptical excision

V-Y flap design in skin creases and left attached to deep tissue

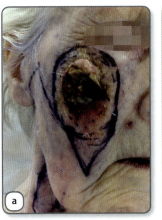

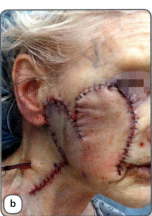

Figure 20.6 (a, b) Fungating squamous cell carcinoma (SCC) on cheek and local bilobed flap.

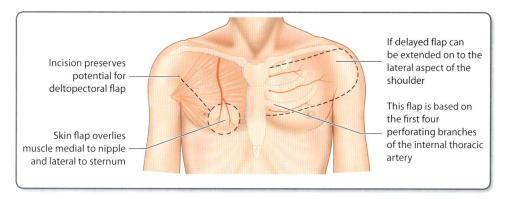

Incision preserves potential for deltopectoral flap

Skin flap overlies muscle medial to nipple and lateral to sternum

If delayed flap can be extended on to the lateral aspect of the shoulder

This flap is based on the first four perforating branches of the internal thoracic artery

Figure 20.7 The pectoralis major and the deltopectoral flap.

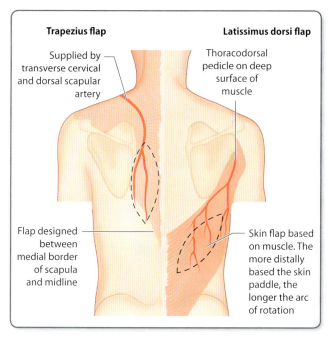

Figure 20.8 The latissimus dorsi and the trapezius myocutaneous flaps.

Trapezius flap

Latissimus dorsi flap

Supplied by transverse cervical and dorsal scapular artery

Thoracodorsal pedicle on deep surface of muscle

Flap designed between medial border of scapula and midline

Skin flap based on muscle. The more distally based the skin paddle, the longer the arc of rotation

myocutaneous flap. The provision of an appropriate one-stage reconstruction is important to avoid problems with scar contracture and to provide tissue that will tolerate radiotherapy when indicated.

Scalp and calvarial defects

Small defects in the skull can often be left with no adverse effects, as long as well covered by soft tissue, but larger defects often require reconstruction for cosmetic purposes and also to protect the brain. The mainstay of calvarial reconstruction is the use of prosthetic

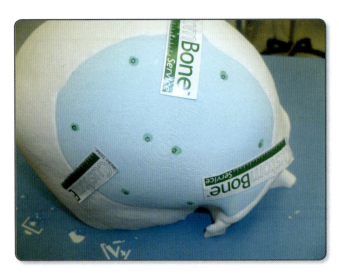

Figure 20.9 Custom made ceramic prosthesis for skull reconstruction made using information from a high resolution CT scan.

materials, methylmethacrylate cement, titanium plates and custom made ceramic prostheses (**Figure 20.9**). Small defects can be closed with calvarial bone graft. Common to all these techniques is the need to cover the calvarial reconstruction with vascularized tissue. What to use depends on the size and site of the defect and the condition of the remaining scalp. Many small to moderate-sized defects can be closed with scalp transposition and rotation flaps, the former usually requiring a skin graft on the donor site. Where the defect is too big or the local tissues are unsuitable a free flap is often required and a muscle only latissimus dorsi with a split skin graft for cover can provide excellent results. An anterolateral thigh flap can also provide a large area of thin pliable tissue. Tissue expansion can be very helpful but as the process takes 6–12 weeks to provide enough excess tissue is not appropriate for use in the immediate reconstructive setting.

Maxillary defects

The reconstructive technique used for maxillary reconstruction will depend on the defect and remains controversial. Many clinicians prefer a dental plate and obturator reconstruction as this allows inspection of the cavity for recurrence. While good functional outcomes are reported with this technique, large defects require more complex reconstructions. The maxilla provides bony support for the midface, the orbital floor and, of course, the alveolar support for the dentition. Brown's classification (**Box 20.1**) assesses both the vertical or surgical defect (1–6) and the horizontal or dental defect (a–d). Small defects can be well managed with obturation. As the defect enlarges retention of an obturator and the stability of a dental prosthesis is more difficult to ensure. The ideal flap reconstruction will provide both hard and soft tissue reconstruction. While pedicled flaps such as temporalis, deltopectoral and buccal fat

Box 20.1 Brown's classification of maxillary defects

Class	Vertical component defect
1	Maxillectomy not causing an oronasal fistula
2	Not involving the orbit
3	Involving the orbital adnexae with orbital retention
4	With orbital enucleation or exenteration
5	Orbitomaxillary defect
6	Nasomaxillary defect
Letter	**Horizontal component defect**
a	Palatal defect only, not dental alveolus
b	≤ ½ of the bilateral or transverse anterior
c	≤ ½ of the unilateral alveolus
d	> ½ of the maxillary alveolus

Table 20.2 Options for maxillary reconstruction

Flap	Advantages	Disadvantages
DCIA	Large reliable bone with muscle	Short pedicle (may require vein grafts) Painful donor site Risk of abdominal hernia
Fibular	Long reliable piece of bone Multiple osteotomies possible Thin pliable skin paddle Muscle can be used for soft tissue reconstruction Minimal donor morbidity	Short bone height can make dental implants unreliable Short bone height unsuitable for maxillary and orbital floor reconstruction
Scapula	Can be harvested as a chimeric flap on the thoracodorsal pedicle with skin paddles and latissimus dorsi, Donor site usually well tolerated	Relatively small piece of bone Requirement to turn patient

flaps have been described, they are unsuitable for extensive defects. Composite free tissue transfer is the mainstay of reconstruction of large defects (**Table 20.2**). The three flaps most commonly used are the deep circumflex iliac artery (DCIA) flap with iliac crest and internal oblique muscle, the fibular osseocutaneous flap and the scapular composite flap.

The ideal reconstruction will provide closure of any oral antral fistula, bony support for the dentition, midface and nose and orbit and a lining for the lateral nasal cavity. For extensive defects (3c–d and 4), the DCIA probably represents the best option.

Mandibular defects

Reconstruction of the mandibular defect is covered in detail in Chapter 15. The ideal reconstruction will provide robust well vascularized bone and sufficient soft tissue to replace resected skin and mucosa. There are three main options and these are the free fibula, the free deep circumflex iliac artery flap and the scapular flap (**Table 20.3**).

Table 20.3 Options for mandibular reconstruction				
Flap	Advantages	Disadvantages	Pedicle length	Bone length
Fibula	Minimal donor morbidity Long pedicle Thin pliable flexible skin paddle Multiple osteotomies possible	Multiple osteotomies may be needed Short bone height	5 cm	25–30 cm
DCIA	Large piece of bone can be cut to match mandibular defect	Painful donor site Short pedicle Risk of abdominal hernia Skin paddle can be unreliable	4–7 cm	15 × 6 cm
Scapula	Thin pliable skin Can be used as chimeric flap on subscapular system	Need to turn patient during procedure	3–7 cm	10 × 2 cm
Pectoralis major	Reliable Can be used when free flaps are contraindicated	Bulky flap Limited arc of rotation	N/a	Variable

Vascularized bone can also be harvested with a free radial forearm flap, but the bone is relatively small and donor site morbidity can be high.

In the edentulous patient reconstruction is relatively simple in that the priority is to maintain the jaw contour and position of the chin point. Osseointegrated implants may be used if there is sufficient bone height in the reconstruction. Where a segmental mandibulectomy is performed in a dentate patient it is of upmost importance to maintain the occlusion of the residual teeth and therefore the reconstruction must accurately reflect the length and contour resected.

The fibular flap has the advantage of low donor site morbidity, the option of simultaneous resection and flap raising and a thin pliable skin paddle. However, careful planning is required as the bone requires osteotomies to provide any contour (**Figure 20.10**). The scapular flap

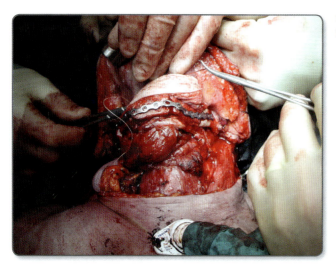

Figure 20.10 Free fibula inset and fixed with a reconstruction plate.

shares the low donor morbidity but has the limitation that the patient must be turned to harvest the flap and this can prolong the procedure. The bone length harvested may also be shorter. The scapular flap may be harvested with one or more (scapular-parascapular) skin flaps and as a chimeric flap with latissimus dorsi and serratus anterior, for example. The DCIA flap provides a large piece of curved bone, which can be shaped to mimic the mandible. However, the donor site is often very painful and can result in abdominal hernias. The pedicle length may be comparatively short.

Fixation of the reconstructed mandible may be with titanium miniplates or a locking reconstruction plate. While each has its perceived advantages and disadvantages, the literature does not identify a significant difference in outcomes.

Defects of floor of mouth and oral tongue

Many small floor of mouth and oral tongue defects may be closed directly or allowed to heal secondarily particularly after laser resection. However if the resection is likely to limit the mobility of the tongue or compromise the integrity of the floor of the mouth a flap reconstruction may be needed. Local flaps such as nasolabial flaps or facial artery myomucosal flaps may be suitable for smaller defects and good results are described. For larger defects then pedicled flaps may be used such as a latissimus dorsi and pectoralis major flap. The former has the disadvantage of requiring the patient to be turned during the procedure but can provide a large reliable flap. The pectoralis major flap is also a reliable reconstruction. However, both flaps can be very bulky and difficult to successfully place into the floor of mouth. Such reconstructions are best reserved for larger defects in patients unsuited to free flap reconstruction.

Larger defects of the floor of mouth and ventral tongue that require lining are best reconstructed using a free radial forearm flap. However for defects of more than half the tongue a larger bulkier flap may be required in the form of an anterolateral thigh (ALT) flap (with or without a section of vastus lateralis) or a rectus abdominis flap.

Total glossectomy is an extremely disabling procedure as not only is the function of the tongue lost but the suspension of the larynx is also destroyed. Functional and non-functional reconstructions have been described. The former, involving the use of sensate flaps, require nerve anastomosis. Results are of dubious value. The most important thing is to provide enough bulk in the oral cavity to enable the food bolus to be propelled posteriorly.

Defects of the oropharynx

The key concerns are to achieve a seal, avoid stricture, maintain velopharyngeal competence and not delay the use of adjuvant therapies if required. Small defects of the oropharynx may be left to spontaneously re-epythelialise with excellent results. The use of robotic surgery has potentially increased the number of surgical defects that can be left to heal secondarily. If larger defects are created, a more complex reconstruction will be required. The ideal reconstruction will provide thin pliable tissue that can be draped over the complex topography of the oropharynx. The free radial forearm flap is an excellent choice. In thin patients, a lateral arm or thinned ALT flap may be appropriate.

Reconstruction of the hypopharynx

Reconstruction of the hypopharynx is challenging and technically demanding. Patients require multimodality treatment and even when managed aggressively have 2-year disease specific survival of around 25%. The key objectives of hypopharyngeal reconstruction are rehabilitation of the patients swallowing and speech. Voice rehabilitation is achieved either by the placement of a speech valve or training the patient in the use of esophageal speech. Both require a pliable flap that is stiff enough to maintain a lumen for an air column to vibrate.

There have been many different reconstructive options described all of which have advantages and disadvantages. As yet, no single reconstructive technique has proven vastly superior to all others (**Table 20.4**). It is important that the reconstructive surgical team have a range of options to tailor to each patient. Complications with these patients may be catastrophic (e.g. mediastinitis) and it is therefore important

Table 20.4 Options for hypopharynx reconstruction		
Flap	**Advantages**	**Disadvantages**
Pectoralis major	Relatively quick	Bulky flap which can be difficult to tube Poor donor site result
Free radial forearm	Thin pliable skin Long pedicle Quick to raise Simultaneous resection and raising	Perception that flap is too thin and pliable Poor donor site for flap of this size Potential for flap failure, especially in the patient with vascular disease, with serious consequences
Free anterolateral thigh flap	Large pliable flap Long pedicle Excellent donor site Low fistula rate Simultaneous resection and raising	Dissection can be unpredictable
Free jejunal Flap	Mucosa to mucosa anastomosis Low fistula rate	Wet voice High stricture rate with postoperative radiotherapy Requires laparotomy, with attendant risks
Gastric pull up	Mucosa to mucosa anastomosis Low fistula rate Will deal with skip lesions lower in oesophagus Single anastomosis	Requires laparotomy and or thoracotomy High complication rate

that the reconstructive surgeon is prepared to deal with these should they occur.

The most commonly used reconstructions are the free radial forearm flap, anterolateral thigh flap, free jejunum and pectoralis major pedicled myocutaneous flap. The monitoring of 'buried' free flaps presents a challenge, as does the protection of the vascular anastomoses, from potential salivary leaks.

A summary of the advantages and disadvantages of the various techniques can be found in **Table 20.4**. The individual choice of reconstruction must be tailored to the individual patient taking many factors into account, including comorbidities, size of defect, and body habitus.

Summary

The development of reliable techniques to reconstruct major head and neck defects allows the resection of large head and neck tumors while optimizing functional and aesthetic outcomes. The literature is unclear in many cases as to which technique is most effective. It is therefore important to have a range of techniques available to the reconstructive surgeon so that the most appropriate one can be selected for the individual patient and the local resources.

Further reading

Brown JS, Rogers SN, McNally DN, Boyle M. A modified classification for the maxillectomy defect. Head Neck 2000; 22:17–26.

Cordeiro PG, Disa JJ, Hidalgo DA, Hu QY. Reconstruction of the mandible with osseous free flaps: a 10 year experience with 150 consecutive patients. Plast Reconstr Surg 1999; 104:1314–20.

Mardini S, Salgado CJ, Kim Evans KF, Chen HC. Reconstruction of the esophagus and voice. Plast Reconstr Surg 2010; 126:471–85.

Miles BA, Goldstein DP, Gilbert RW, Gullane PJ. Mandible reconstruction. Curr Opin Otolaryngol Head Neck Surg 2010; 18:317–22.

Murray DJ, Novak CB, Neligan PC. Fasciocutaneous free flaps in pharyngolaryngo-oesophageal reconstruction: a critical review of the literature. J Plast Reconstr Aesthet Surg 2008; 61:1148–56.

Robey AB, Spann ML, McAuliff TM, et al. Comparison of miniplates and reconstruction plates in fibular flap reconstruction of the mandible. Plast Reconstr Surg 2008; 122:1733–8.

Wei FC, Dayan JH. Scalp, skull, orbit and maxilla construction and hair transplantation. Plast Reconstr Surg 2013; 131:411e–24e.

Index

Note: Page numbers in **bold** or *italic* refer to tables or figures, respectively.